Preventive Cardiology: How can we reduce CVD risk?

Harald M Lipman (Ed.)
Joe Rosenthal
Tamar Koch Richard Meakin

# Preventive Cardiology: How can we reduce CVD risk?

## Reducing Cardiovascular Disease Risk

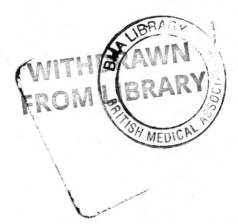

**LAP LAMBERT Academic Publishing**

## Impressum / Imprint

Bibliografische Information der Deutschen Nationalbibliothek: Die Deutsche Nationalbibliothek verzeichnet diese Publikation in der Deutschen Nationalbibliografie; detaillierte bibliografische Daten sind im Internet über http://dnb.d-nb.de abrufbar.

Alle in diesem Buch genannten Marken und Produktnamen unterliegen warenzeichen-, marken- oder patentrechtlichem Schutz bzw. sind Warenzeichen oder eingetragene Warenzeichen der jeweiligen Inhaber. Die Wiedergabe von Marken, Produktnamen, Gebrauchsnamen, Handelsnamen, Warenbezeichnungen u.s.w. in diesem Werk berechtigt auch ohne besondere Kennzeichnung nicht zu der Annahme, dass solche Namen im Sinne der Warenzeichen- und Markenschutzgesetzgebung als frei zu betrachten wären und daher von jedermann benutzt werden dürften.

Bibliographic information published by the Deutsche Nationalbibliothek: The Deutsche Nationalbibliothek lists this publication in the Deutsche Nationalbibliografie; detailed bibliographic data are available in the Internet at http://dnb.d-nb.de.

Any brand names and product names mentioned in this book are subject to trademark, brand or patent protection and are trademarks or registered trademarks of their respective holders. The use of brand names, product names, common names, trade names, product descriptions etc. even without a particular marking in this work is in no way to be construed to mean that such names may be regarded as unrestricted in respect of trademark and brand protection legislation and could thus be used by anyone.

Coverbild / Cover image: www.ingimage.com

Verlag / Publisher:
LAP LAMBERT Academic Publishing
ist ein Imprint der / is a trademark of
OmniScriptum GmbH & Co. KG
Bahnhofstraße 28, 66111 Saarbrücken, Deutschland / Germany
Email: info@lap-publishing.com

Herstellung: siehe letzte Seite /
Printed at: see last page
ISBN: 978-3-659-79797-2

# Preventive Cardiology: How can we reduce risk?

Editor

Dr Harald M Lipman

*Executive Director International Cardiac Healthcare & RiskFactor Modification (ICHARM)*

*formerly Senior Medical Adviser Foreign & Commonwealth Office*

Authors

Dr Joe Rosenthal

*Senior Lecturer*

*Department of Primary Care & Population Health*

*UCL Medical School*

Dr Richard Meakin

*Senior Clinical Lecturer*

*Department of Primary Care & Population Health*

*UCL Medical School*

Dr Tamar Koch

*Senior Clinical Research Associate*

*Department of Primary Care & Population Health*

*UCL Medical School*

This manual is based on a training course devised and taught by ICHARM in Bashkortostan Republic Russia

The following copyright permissions have been granted:

WHO CVD mortality. Prevalence of tobacco use in Russia & England

Professor Paul Durrington    JBS2

OUP HeartScore charts

ClinRisk Ltd QRISK2 chart

Professor Karl Fagerström    Fagerström Test

Dr Neil Chapman    Case studies

ONS    Cigarette smokers in UK

NCBI    AUDIT-C test

NHS    Motivation to stop smoking. Smoking motives questionnaire. General Practice Physical Activity Questionnaire

British Heart Foundation    Burden of CVD in UK

OECD    Life expectancy at birth

Statista   Prevalence of raised BP in selected countries

American Institute of Stress    Holmes-Rahe Stress Inventory

NICE Management of type 2 diabetes 2015    Management of primary hypertension CG 127

Alcohol Education Trust Units in a Drink

ABPI    Interplay of factors in development of atheroma

## Contents

# Foreword

Cardiovascular diseases are major causes of death and disability and, in 2012 were responsible for 17.5 million deaths worldwide. They are driven by the effects of globalization on marketing and trade, rapid unplanned urbanization and ageing of populations. A large number of deaths due to cardiovascular diseases are premature, under the age of 70 years and are highly preventable. For instance, in 2012, cardiovascular diseases were responsible for the largest proportion (37%) of non-communicable disease deaths (16 million), under the age of 70 years. A combination of multisectoral, population wide strategies and individual based strategies is essential for prevention of cardiovascular diseases. In this context it is a pleasure to introduce this manual on **preventive cardiology behaviour and lifestyle modification**. It focuses mainly on prevention of cardiovascular disease at the individual level.

The manual provides information on the magnitude and causes of cardiovascular disease, ways of detecting people at risk of developing cardiovascular events and preventing them by modifying the risk using lifestyle modification and appropriate medication. Useful information is provided on how to assess the cardiovascular risk of individuals, what advice to give to help them to modify risk behaviours and what treatments are available to reduce the chances of developing cardiovascular disease in the future.

Health professionals, particularly those working at primary care level have a vital role to play in prevention of cardiovascular disease at individual level. They need to possess a sound knowledge in cardiovascular health to perform this role effectively. The manual is relevant and germane because it highlights what can be done by health workers to improve cardiovascular health of individuals. It is written in a style which is easy to understand. A chapter is devoted to each key area of cardiovascular prevention. Each chapter provides some information as well as opportunities to discuss cases with colleagues or try out new ways of communicating with patients.

The target audience of this manual are primary care physicians, practice nurses, junior hospital doctors in the fields of Cardiology and Public Heath, dieticians, physiotherapists, physical trainers and social workers in the United Kingdom. With appropriate amendments and translations it could also serve as a useful resource for training of health workers in preventive cardiology worldwide.

*Professor Shanthi Mendis MBBS, MD, FRCP, FACC*
*WHO Global Coordinator Prevention & Management of Non-Communicable Diseases*

# Introduction

Welcome to the ICHARM Cardiovascular Disease (CVD) Prevention manual. Thank you for taking the time out from your busy lives to learn about CVD prevention – why it is important, and what you can do to help people improve their CVD health.

The importance of teaching preventive cardiology in the UK is highlighted in a recent paper assessing management of CVD prevention in General Practice in the UK which showed that only one third of all patients studied received optimal advice and treatment.

What is preventive cardiology? The art and science of recognising and managing individuals at high risk of developing CVD, in order to reduce their risk by lifestyle modification and use of appropriate medication.

The aims of this manual are to remind you about the causes of CVD, to place the condition in epidemiological context by exploring how large a problem CVD is worldwide and to demonstrate ways of reducing this enormous problem.

Firstly, we look at some global epidemiological data with particular emphasis on cardiovascular mortality, comparing UK with other countries, taking Russia, as an example of an upper middle income country (Appendix A).

Next we briefly consider the issue of health inequalities and social determinants of health, a topical subject which has recently been recognised and which has been shown to be linked to poorer population outcomes.

We remind ourselves of the basic cardiac anatomy and physiology (Appendix B), the pathophysiology of CVD and its effect on other organs in the body (Appendix C).

We will be showing in more detail why CVD prevention is relevant to the public and all health professionals. We will revise what CVD is, how it causes mortality and morbidity, how it can be prevented by addressing lifestyle and medical factors, and how in particular you as primary care physicians have a huge role to play in helping prevention of CVD.

How can we help people to change their behaviour and encourage them to modify their lifestyles?

There are lifestyle risk factors which increase the risk of developing CVD which can be explored with each individual patient. In addition, there are ways to determine who is at high risk of developing CVD and there are modifications which those people at high risk can make in order to reduce their chances of developing CVD. Modifications in terms of medications and simultaneously in terms of lifestyle behaviours. We show you how to assess individuals, what advice to give, and what treatments are available in order to help your patients reduce their chances of developing CVD in the future.

We consider the management of related or causative medical problems. We discuss high risk populations, cost effective prevention strategies, hard to reach populations, incentive schemes and finally we show you how to plan and introduce preventive cardiology programmes.

In parallel at a population level we detail measures which can be taken by nations and governments to reduce the mortality and morbidity rate of this important health problem.

The long term aim is to reduce the huge burden of CVD in the UK, Europe and Worldwide in both developed and developing countries.

Remember - CVD is a major cause of morbidity and mortality worldwide within the modality of non-communicable diseases. This causes widespread illness and social and economic loss to both the individual and society.

Non-communicable diseases (NCDs) have become the primary health concern for most countries around the world. Currently, more than 38 million people worldwide die from NCDs each year, accounting for 63% of annual global deaths; over 40% of these are preventable. 82% of NCD global deaths occur in low- and middle-income countries. The global financial burden of NCDs is staggering, with an estimated 2010, global cost of US$6.3 trillion (£4.2 trillion) that is projected to increase to US$13 trillion (£8.7 trillion) by 2030.

A number of NCDs, including CVD, cancer of lung, stomach, colon and possibly breast, diabetes and chronic respiratory disease (COPD) share one or more common predisposing risk factors, all related to lifestyle to some degree.

**References:**

➤ Healthy lifestyle interventions to combat non-communicable disease - a novel non-hierarchical connectivity model for key stakeholders: a policy statement from the American Heart Association, European Society of Cardiology, European Association for Cardiovascular Prevention and Rehabilitation, and American College of Preventive Medicine Eur Heart J 2015 36: 2097-2109

➤ WHO Global status report on-communicable disease 2014

➤ Sheppard Missed opportunities in prevention of CVD in primary care Br J Gen Pract 2014; 64:28-29

# 1. The Global Problem of Cardiovascular Disease (CVD)

## Key Points

- CVD deaths are the number 1 cause of death globally.
- CVD is the biggest killer of women globally.
- The developing countries contribute a greater share to the global burden of CVD than the developed countries.
- Most deaths are avoidable, by targeting risk factors such as smoking, alcohol, obesity, physical inactivity, stress, hypertension, diabetes and raised lipids.

## 1.1 CVD Globally

To demonstrate the global nature of the problem of CVD and compare similarities and differences in the presentation and management of the problem we shall show the situation in England and that in Scotland and the Russian Federation (see Appendix A).

Let us remind you why CVD prevention is important globally and what you can do to help with this massive disease burden.

- More people die each year in the world from CVD than from any other cause. In 2012, an estimated 17.5 million people died from CVD globally – this represents 31% of all deaths.
- 7.4 million are due to Coronary heart disease (CHD), 6.7 million due to Stroke. Over three quarters of these occur in low- and middle-income countries.

Perhaps even more importantly, every year 20 million people worldwide survive heart attacks and strokes and many of these require costly clinical care.

- In Europe 47% of deaths in men and women are due to CVD, accounting for 4 million deaths annually. In 28 of the 49 European countries, including Finland, Greece and the UK, CVD is the main cause of death in men aged less than 65 years.

- Compare this with the situation in the Russian Federation. CVD is responsible for 51% of all deaths and largely due to this until 2010 the Russian population was falling annually by 0.5%.

- Within the UK, as in many countries, there is considerable regional variation. In Scotland the death rate from CVD for men is 50% higher than in South West England. The highest death rates are found in the West of Scotland.

- In Europe 61 million years of healthy life, disability adjusted life years (DALYs), are lost annually, due to CVD, of which 11 million are in the EU. In 2014 the EU lost the equivalent of £102 billion (€81 billion, US$153 billion), based on lost years of healthy life (DALYs), due to CVD and related illness (0.8% of total GDP).

- The developing countries contribute a greater share to the global burden of CVD than the developed countries. More than 75% of deaths from CVD occur in low- and middle-income countries.

- Most deaths are avoidable, by targeting risk factors such as smoking, alcohol, obesity, physical inactivity, hypertension, diabetes and raised lipids.
- Reduction of CVD can be achieved through improving public awareness and by targeted health interventions.

**References:**

➤ http://www.who.int/mediacentre/factsheets/fs317/en/index.html 2015
➤ Global Atlas of Cardiovascular Diseases Prevention & Control WHO 2011
➤ European CVD Statistics European Society of Cardiology 2012
➤ National Statistics Publication for Scotland Heart Disease Statistics 2014
➤ Economic costs of CVD from 2014-2020 in 6 European economies Cebr 2014
➤ World Bank Data Catalog (European Union) 2015
➤ WHO Media Centre Cardiovascular Diseases Jan 2015

## 1.2 CVD in the UK

- CVD accounts for approximately 155,000 deaths in the UK (1/4 of all deaths).
- 38,000 male and 27,000 female deaths occur annually due to CHD.
- In the last 30 years deaths in the UK from CVD have been reduced by 68%.

**Reference:**

➤ British Heart Foundation Headline Statistics 2015

### 1.2.1 Demographic Data for England

- In 2007 in England there were >100,000 heart attacks, 62,000 in men and 39,000 in women.
- In 2010 more than 65,000 people died from Coronary Heart Disease (CHD) in England.
- In 2008 CVD caused 28% of premature deaths in men under 75 years of age.
- Mortality rates from CVD are 50% higher in the most deprived fifth of the population, than in the least deprived one-fifth.
- In 2007 57,000 men and 68,000 women suffered strokes.

**Reference:**

➢ British Heart Foundation Coronary Heart Disease Statistics 2012

### 1.2.2 Demographic Data for Scotland

- In 2010 there were 17,000 deaths from CVD in Scotland. One third of total deaths (total population 5,295,000 census 2011).
- 12,000 people had heart attacks. 7,000 men and 5,000 women. 270,000 people had CHD and 200,000 suffer angina.
- In 2013 approximately 8,000 deaths were due to CHD.
- Premature mortality rates are 25% higher in Scotland than in England.
- CHD age and sex standardised incidence rate decreased by 27.3% between 2003 and 2012.

5

**Reference:**

- ➤ British Heart Foundation CHD Statistics in Scotland 2012
- ➤ National Statistics Publication for Scotland Heart Disease Statistics 2014

## 1.3 Life Expectancy at Birth 1970 to 2011

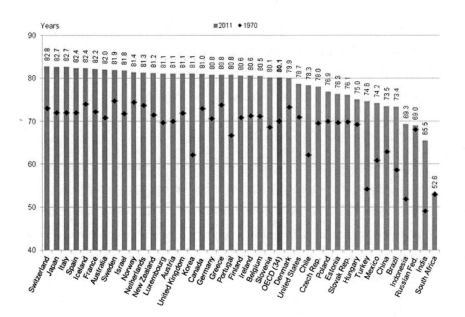

### 1.3.1 Life Expectancy in Europe

There is wide variation in life expectancy amongst many countries and in most countries life expectation increased over the period 1970 to 2011. Whilst other European countries developed in a way which resulted in an increase in life expectancy, the life expectancy in countries such as Russia actually dropped during the 40 years.

From 1945 to 1960 mortality improved considerably in the eastern region of Europe because of improvements in housing and hygiene, and the control of communicable diseases. At that time there was only a small discrepancy between life expectancy in eastern and western countries of Europe.

By the 1970s and 1980s life expectancy in Western Europe started to significantly improve because of work and lifestyle modification and reduction in deaths from non-communicable diseases, but this was not so in Eastern Europe, leading to a wider gap between the two regions. Since 2010 there has been a small reduction in early mortality from heart disease in Russia and an increase in life expectancy.

Much of the reduction in life expectancy was related to lifestyle factors, such as poor diet, inadequate physical activity, excessive smoking and alcohol consumption and increased levels of stress. All these factors leading to increased CVD and other smoking- and alcohol-related diseases. Accidents and injuries further contributed to the reduced life expectancy.

**References:**

➢ OECD Health database 2015

  http://stats.oecd.org/index.aspx?DataSetCode=HEALTH_STAT

➢ WHO Statistical Information System (WHOSIS) 2013

  http://www.who.int/whosis/en/; European Health Expectancy

➢ Monitoring Unit: http://www.ehemu.eu/; and, Mathers C.D., Murray C.J., and Samson J. (2003) Methods for Measuring

In 2006 for men in the UK life expectancy at birth was 74 years, not far different from Chinese men who had a life expectancy at birth of 72 years. British women at birth could expect to live to an average age of 78, compared to 73 for women in Russia. The rates in India were similar to those in the Russian Federation, but their lives were cut short more often for different reasons. In India, as well as having high rates of non-communicable diseases, poor living, poor housing and poor hygiene conditions mean that there is a higher prevalence of communicable diseases, which additionally accounts for more deaths.

A boy born in 2012 in a high-income country can expect to live to the age of around 76. 16 years longer than a boy born in a low-income country (age at death 60). For girls, the difference is even wider as a gap of 19 years separates life expectancy in high-income (82 years) and low-income countries (63 years).

**References:**

➢ Global Health Observatory (GHO) 2014 WHO

  http://www.who.int/gho/mortality_burden_disease/life_tables/hale/en

➢ World Health Statistics 2014

## 1.4 Global Mortality from CVD

WHO data from 2012 of death rates from CVD per 100,000 population in both sexes, worldwide, including CVD deaths related to diabetes, showed a very high rate in the Russian Federation and the whole of the Eastern European block, in comparison with Western European countries and North American and even much of Asia.

Most deaths which result from diabetes occur because of micro- and macro-vascular damage to vessels from the free glucose in the blood (this occurs in diabetes). So although the pathology results from glycaemia, the actual mode of death is cardiovascular.

The values were standardized for age. Standardisation of ages is a statistical technique used to ensure comparisons of different populations are accurate and relevant. In other words, some populations, for example, may have a larger proportion of elderly, which would result in a proportionately higher rate of CVD deaths, compared to a population with a larger proportion of young people (because older people are more likely to have developed CVD). Age standardisation takes these differences into account, so that the populations are comparable.

Data from 72 countries showed that CVD and diabetes mortality was more concentrated in middle- and low-income countries and was negatively associated with GDP, GINI index (a measure of inequality of wealth amongst nations), and western diet. Countries with high average blood pressure had higher mortality rates showing a positive relationship.

**Reference:**

➢ Zahra A et al Cardiovascular disease and diabetes mortality, and their relation to socio-economical, environmental, and health behavioural factors in worldwide view. The Royal Society for Public Health April 2015 Volume 129, Issue 4, Pages 385–395

## 1.5 Heart Disease in Women

- CVD is the biggest killer of women globally. Annually worldwide 8.6 million women die from heart disease and stroke, (one third of all female deaths).

- Women in low- and middle-income countries who develop CVD are more likely to die from it than women in industrialized nations and have a higher proportion of CVD deaths than men in those countries.

- Women with diabetes have higher CVD mortality rates than men with diabetes.

- Risk factors for men and women are largely similar. Women who smoke double their risk of stroke. Women who are obese increase their risk of CHD by 2.48 times. Women with hypertension have a 3.5 times risk compared with normotensive women.

**Reference:**

➢ Cardiovascular disease in women Fact sheet World Heart Federation 2012

## 1.6 Ethnic Differences in CVD in the UK

- Compared with the general population in the UK incidence of myocardial infarct is higher in South Asians.
- Incidence of stroke is higher in Black ethnic groups.
- Incidence of CHD is higher in those born in India and Pakistan.
- Diabetes incidence is higher in black Caribbeans, Indians, Pakistani and Bangladeshi.
- Binge drinking is lower in all ethnic minority groups.
- BMI is lower in South Asians and Chinese.
- Overweight and obesity has a higher incidence in black children.

**Reference:**

➢ British Heart Foundation 2010 Ethnic Differences in Cardiovascular Disease

## In Summary

Have we met the objectives?

- To highlight the global nature and prevalence of CVD in the UK and Worldwide.
- To become familiar with the epidemiology of CVD globally and nationally, to be able to give an example of a country with low rates of CVD and a country with high rates.

Remember - CVD is a major cause of morbidity and mortality worldwide within the modality of non-communicable diseases. This causes widespread illness and social and economic loss to both the individual and society.

# Preventive Cardiology

## 2. CVD and Prevention

### Key Points

- There are major inequalities in health both between countries globally, and even within each country.
- Changing peoples' health-related behaviour can have a major impact on some of the causes of mortality and morbidity including CVD.

### 2.1 What you already know about CVD and its Prevention

Before we launch into the information-giving part of this chapter let us look at what you already know about the topic of preventive medicine, CVD and cardiovascular prevention.

What is your definition of CVD?

The World Health Organisation (WHO) defines it as *"a group of disorders of the heart and blood vessels which include Coronary Heart Disease, Cerebrovascular Disease, Peripheral Arterial Disease, Rheumatic Heart Disease, Congenital Heart Disease and Deep Vein Thrombosis/Pulmonary Embolic Disease."*

*Why is CVD so important to today's society?*
*Why is it relevant to health practitioners in the UK and worldwide?*
*What do we know about preventive medicine?*
*What are the differences between primary, secondary, and tertiary prevention?*

**Primary prevention**, the first level of healthcare, is designed to prevent the occurrence of a disease and promote health.

Examples of primary prevention are hand washing, immunisations, barrier contraception, smoking cessation.

**Secondary prevention**, the second level of healthcare, is designed to identify conditions which can lead to diseases or to identify diseases in their earliest manifestations, in order to limit complications and negative sequelae.

Examples of secondary prevention are cervical screening, mammography, blood pressure monitoring, antenatal monitoring.

**Tertiary prevention**, the third level of healthcare, is designed to promote independent function and reduce further morbidity or mortality once a disease has been active.

Examples of tertiary prevention are regular eye checks for diabetic patients, regular colonoscopies for patients with colonic polyps, regular imaging for people who have been treated for cancer.

Do you already practise any cardiovascular preventive assessments/measures with your patients?

In subsequent chapters we shall be looking at all these specific matters in greater detail.

For the moment let us concentrate on the effect of certain relevant determinants of healthcare and ways of creating beneficial changes.

**Reference:**

➢ At Work, Issue 80, Spring 2015: Institute for Work & Health, Toronto

## 2.2 Health Inequalities and Social Determinants of Health

There are major inequalities in health both between countries globally, and even within each country – this has been shown throughout the world, in countries such as USA, UK and the Netherlands. We now know that these inequalities arise from inequalities in social determinants of health.

Social determinants of health are the economic and social conditions - and their distribution in society - which influence individual and group differences in health status. The conditions in which a person is born, grows, lives, works and ages are shaped by the distribution of money, power, and resources (including the health system) at the macro- (global), meso- (national) and micro- (local) levels. These include economic situations, educational strategy and social welfare programmes.

The disproportionately unequal division of these modalities leads to avoidable inequities in health both between and even within countries. The lower someone's social position in society, the worse his/her health is likely to be. Social and economic conditions can prevent people from changing their behaviour to improve their health and can also reinforce behaviours that damage it.

This disproportionate or unequal distribution of power, money or resources, may affect the health of the population you are responsible for. Thus some of the 'choices' people make, are not necessarily under their control, but are a product of the environment in which – often unfairly and avoidably – they find themselves.

**Reference:**

> ➤ Behaviour changes: the principles for effective interventions NICE Public Health guidance 6 2007

Unquestionably the way we think and live plays a large part in influencing our health. What can be done to alter and improve the situation?

## 2.3 Changing Behaviour and Lifestyle Modification

Changing peoples' health-related behaviour can have a major impact on some of the causes of mortality and morbidity including CVD. Different patterns of behaviour are deeply embedded in peoples' social and material circumstances and their cultural context.

Interventions to change behaviour have enormous potential to alter current patterns of disease.

Behaviour change may be delivered at individual, household, community or population levels. Cognitive-behavioural methods are effective in supporting persons in adopting a healthier lifestyle.

Significant events or transition points in peoples' lives, such as leaving school, starting work, becoming a parent, becoming unemployed, retirement and bereavement present important opportunities to intervene.

**References:**

> ➤ Behaviour change NICE PH6 2007 www.nice.org.uk/PH6
> ➤ Abraham & Mitchie Theoretical frameworks for behaviour change Health Psychology 2008 27, (3): 379-387
> ➤ ESC guidelines on cardiovascular disease prevention in clinical practice 2012

## 2.4 Assessing Readiness for Change
### 2.4.1 Cycle of Change

Pre contemplation-Contemplation-Preparation-Action-Maintenance.

Sometimes, even though you make a persuasive argument for someone's behaviour to change they are not ready to make changes.

Di Clementi's 'Cycle of Change' shows the stages a person goes through as part of changing behaviour. At first, she/he may not be ready to even think about changing – this is the **pre-contemplation** stage. At this stage, if somebody is explicit about not wanting or being ready to even think about changing their behaviour, the best you can do as a health practitioner is to try to find out what reasons she/he gives for not wanting to change and just listening, rather than giving direct instructions contradicting them or their readiness to change. The other very important role a clinician has at this stage is to offer information about the benefits of changing (especially the health benefits, but also other benefits for example, financial), and the disadvantages of not changing. Once you've given that information and the patient understands, you may just have to leave it at that, and re-visit the topic the next time you meet.

An individual at the **contemplation** stage of change may already be agreeing that they ought to change their health behaviour, for example of drinking excessive amounts of alcohol. At this stage, you can offer information again about the advantages and disadvantages, and you can discuss between you what precise practical changes can be made, and consider setting some goals.

The **preparation** stage is when the individual goes away and gets ready to change, perhaps setting themselves a date when the new behaviour is going to start, and maybe informing their friends and family about the changes they are going to make.

**Action** is making the change and **maintenance** is continuing with the change. An individual may require some support from a health care professional at regular intervals initially, so that you can review the goals and offer support and encouragements.

If an individual relapses back to their unhealthy behaviour, then they enter the cycle all over again.

Whilst this model has its flaws, it can be useful to think about it when interviewing your patients. Where are they on the cycle of change?

This will influence how you respond to them – whether you will simply offer information, or have a more detailed conversation about what changes they can make, and how they can make them.

**Reference:**

➢ Prochaska & Di Clemente The Transtheoretical Model (TTM) approach Handbook of psychotherapy integration OUP 2005 147-171

## 2.4.2 Processes of Change

Strategies that can help people make and maintain change - the TTM calls these *processes of change*. The ten processes include:

*Consciousness Raising* - increasing awareness via information, education, and personal feedback about the healthy behaviour.

*Dramatic Relief* - feeling fear, anxiety, or worry because of the unhealthy behaviour, or feeling inspiration and hope when they hear about how people are able to change to healthy behaviours.

*Self-Re-evaluation* - realizing that the healthy behaviour is an important part of who they are and want to be.

*Environmental Re-evaluation* - realizing how their unhealthy behaviour affects others and how they could have more positive effects by changing.

*Social Liberation* - realizing that society is more supportive of the healthy behaviour.

*Self-Liberation* - believing in one's ability to change and making commitments to act on that belief.

*Helping Relationships* - finding people who are supportive of their change.

*Counter Conditioning* - substituting healthy ways of acting and thinking for unhealthy ways.

*Reinforcement Management* - increasing the rewards that come from positive behaviour and reducing those that come from negative behaviour.

*Stimulus Control* - using reminders and cues that encourage healthy behaviour.

## Summary

- We have studied some of the are major inequalities in health between countries globally, and within each country.
- We have shown how changing peoples' health-related behaviour can have a major impact on some of the causes of CVD mortality and morbidity.

# 3. Cardiovascular Risk Factors and Primary Prevention

## Key Point

- Primary prevention of CVD requires the assessment of individual cardiac risk and introduction of measures to change behaviour and modify existing lifestyle factors.

## Objectives:

- To be able to list nine modifiable and four non-modifiable cardiovascular risk factors.
- To reflect on which risk factors, if any, you address in your practice.
- To begin to stratify patients as high risk or low risk based on clinical presentations in case vignettes.
- To consider particular local issues in the UK.

## 3.1 Risk Factors

Let us first identify the non-modifiable and modifiable risk factors for CVD. We will then go on to look in detail at modifiable risk factors.

Then we will consider a number of case vignettes and use these to begin to categorise these patients in to high and low risk for CVD on the basis of the patient's medical history and examination.

At the end of the chapter we consider CVD in the UK and how as clinicians you may respond to this challenge in your own practice.

### 3.1.1 Non-modifiable Risk Factors

There are a number of risk factors for CVD which are not modifiable.

- **Age**: Risk increases with increasing age.
- **Gender**: Men are at greater risk than pre-menopausal women. After the menopause womens' risk becomes similar to mens'.
- **Family history**: If a first degree blood relative, below the age of 55 years for men and 65 years for women, has or had CVD then that person has an increased risk.
- **Ethnic origin**: People of Asian and African ancestry are at greater risk than other racial groups.

### 3.1.2 Modifiable Risk Factors

- Tobacco use
- Excessive Alcohol consumption
- Unhealthy Diet / Obesity
- Physical inactivity
- Stress
- Hypertension
- Raised Cholesterol
- Diabetes

Having considered those risk factors which neither patients nor their physicians can do anything about, we now consider those which can be modified either by pharmaceutical intervention by physicians or by lifestyle modification by patients. Let us now consider each of these in turn. In later chapters we shall study each risk factor in depth.

**Reference:**

➢ Global Atlas on Cardiovascular Disease Prevention and Control. Mendis S, Puska P, Norrving B editors. World Health Organization (in collaboration with the World Heart Federation and World Stroke Organization), Geneva 2011.

### 3.1.2.1 Tobacco Use - chapter 5

Tobacco use is a major risk factor for CVD as well as being related to development of various cancers. All forms of tobacco use are associated with an increase in CVD. However, smoking is the commonest form of tobacco use. It has been estimated that smoking increases a person's risk of developing CVD by 100% compared to non-smokers.

- Smoking, using snuff and chewing tobacco, all increase the risk of developing CVD.
- The smoke inhaled during one session of shisha smoking is equivalent to smoking at least 50 cigarettes.
- Every day 12 million cigarettes per minute are smoked worldwide.
- In the UK (total population 63 million) 10,000,000 people smoke every day. 21% of men and 20% of women over the age of 18 years smoke.
- In 1974 27% smokers had quit, by 2013 this had risen to 54%.
- The risk is dose dependant in as much as it increases with the amount smoked and the length of time a person smokes.

**References:**

➤ NHS Statistics on smoking, England 2012

➤ ASH Fact sheet July 2012 and 2015 Smoking statistics

➤ Waterpipe Tobacco Smoking: An Emerging Health Crisis in the United States Cobb et al Am J Health Behav. 2010 May-Jun; 34(3): 275–285

### 3.1.2.2 Alcohol Consumption - chapter 6

Alcohol consumption is a risk factor for CVD and consumption of more than 8 units/day (4 pints of beer, 200ml of Whisky/Vodka) is associated with double the risk of CVD in men. The risk is also increased for women. Those women who drink more than 6 units a day increase their risk of developing coronary heart disease by a factor of 1.3 times.

- In the UK in 2011 average alcohol consumption was 10 litres per year (men drank twice as much as women), equivalent to 500 pints of beer.

- Sporadic heavy drinking or 'binge drinking' has a direct toxic effect on the myocardium and is associated with an increased risk of CVD. There is no internationally agreed definition of what constitutes 'binge drinking'. In the UK it is often defined as drinking more than 8 units over a short period of time with the intention of becoming rapidly intoxicated. Another definition is consumption in 1 hour of 0.5 litre or more of 40% alcohol, without food.

- In 2013 21% of UK population drank no alcohol compared with 19% in 2005. In the same period binge drinking had fallen from 18% to 15%.

**References:**

➤ Alcohol consumption Fact Sheet 2013 Institute of Alcohol Studies

➤ Statistics on Alcohol England 2015 Health & Social Care Information Centre

### 3.1.2.3 Unhealthy Diet - chapter 7

An unhealthy diet is one with:

- High Saturated Fat Content
- High Refined Sugar Content
- High Sodium Content

Sodium is often included as a risk factor as it contributes to high levels of LDL–Cholesterol, Obesity and Hypertension.

**Reference:**

➤ European Heart Network. Diet, Physical Activity and Cardiovascular Disease Prevention in Europe 2011

### 3.1.2.4 Obesity - chapter 7

Obesity is a growing health concern in the developed world.

Obesity is usually measured by a person's Body Mass Index (BMI). This is defined as the weight in kilograms divided by the height squared. If a person's BMI is greater than 25 they are considered overweight. Being overweight is associated with other cardiovascular risk factors including hypertension and diabetes mellitus. It is also associated with increased atherosclerosis. These conditions will put them at high risk of developing CVD.

If a patient's BMI is greater than 30 they are obese and at serious risk of CVD.

**Reference:**

> ➢ Berrington de Gonzalez Body-mass index and mortality among 1.46 million white adults N Engl J Med 2010:363: 2211-2219

### 3.1.2.5 Physical Inactivity - chapter 8

Physical activity is important for cardiovascular health. If a person does not engage in regular physical activity the risks to cardiovascular health are similar to those associated with hypertension, high cholesterol and obesity.

Physical activity does not need to be vigorous exercise to have the protective benefit. Studies have shown that 2 hours of moderate activity per week will reduce the risk of CVD by 30%.

There are beneficial effects of physical activity even in patients with existing cardiovascular risk factors. If people keep active evidence suggests that this may lower their risk of premature death compared to inactive people with no risk factors for CVD.

**Reference:**

> ➢ Talbot Changes in leisure time physical activity and risk of all-cause mortality in men and women: the Baltimore Longitudinal Study of Ageing Prev Med 2007:45:169-17

### 3.1.2.6 Stress - chapter 9

The stresses of life have long been thought to increase a person's risk of CVD or a serious coronary or cerebral event. But it is not universally agreed which type of stress causes heart disease.

**Reference:**
> ➢ Whalley Psychological interventions for coronary heart disease Cochrane Database Syst Rev 2011:8; C002902

### 3.1.2.7 Hypertension - chapter 10

Raised blood pressure is also a major risk factor for CVD. The risk increases with increasing blood pressure in all age groups. Treatment of hypertension decreases the risk of CVD.

A statistical measure called a hazard ratio is used to measure risk. A hazard ratio is the ratio of the rate at which an event occurs in one group compared to another.

**Reference:**
> ➢ MacMahon. Blood pressure, stroke and coronary heart disease Lancet 1990:335:765-774

### 3.1.2.8 Cholesterol - chapter 11

A further major risk factor for CVD is the level of cholesterol in the blood. Risk of developing CVD increases with increasing total cholesterol levels.

Cholesterol is carried in the blood in two main forms. LDL-cholesterol, that is cholesterol carried on low density lipoproteins, and HDL-cholesterol, that is carried on high density lipoproteins. The risk of CVD associated with cholesterol is more closely related to the level of LDL-cholesterol in the blood. HDL-cholesterol carries cholesterol away from the blood stream so it does not contribute in the same way to development of atheroma. Higher levels of HDL-cholesterol are therefore associated with lower risk.

Studies suggest that the optimal level of total cholesterol should be less than 5 mmol/l, the optimal level of LDL-cholesterol 3.0 mmol/l or less and the optimal level of HDL-cholesterol should be greater than 1.2 mmol/l in men and greater than 1.0 mmol/l in women.

**Reference:**

➢ Neaton. Serum cholesterol level mortality findings for men screened in the Multiple Risk Factor Intervention trial Arch Intern Med 1992:152:1490-1500

### 3.1.2.9 Diabetes Mellitus - chapter 12

People who develop diabetes are at increased risk of CVD and CVD is the leading cause of death among people with diabetes.

People who have diabetes are two to four times more likely to develop CVD than people without diabetes.

If patients control their blood sugar they can reduce their risk by between 33% to 50%.

**Reference:**

➢ Ray Effect of intensive control of glucose on cardiovascular outcomes and death in patients with diabetes mellitus: a meta-analysis of randomised controlled trials Lancet 2009:373:1765-1772

### 3.1.2.10 Inflammatory Gum Disease and CVD

There appears to be an epidemiological association between periodontitis and CVD, particularly in younger men.

**Reference:**

> Dietrich The epidemiological evidence behind the association between periodontitis and incident atherosclerotic CVD J Clin Periodontol 2013; 40(S14):70-84

### 3.1.2.11 Air Pollution and increased risk of Myocardial Infarct

Studies over many years show a relationship between air pollution, particularly from automobile exhaust, and increased risk of myocardial infarct.

**Reference:**

> Gardener et al Ambient fine particulate air pollution triggers ST elevation myocardial infarction, but not non- ST elevation myocardial infarction Particle & Fibre Toxicology 2014,11:1

### 3.1.2.12 Long Working Hours

Employees who work long hours have an increased risk of stroke.

**Reference:**

> Kivimäki M et al Long working hours and risk of coronary heart disease and stroke: a systematic review and meta-analysis of published and unpublished data for 603 838 individuals 2015 http://dx.doi.org/10.1016/S0140-6736(15)60295-1

## 3.2 Interaction of Multiple Risk Factors

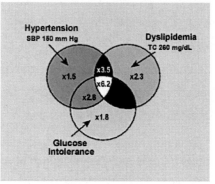

### Risk Factors interact to multiply risk

Multiple risk factors interact to increase the risk of developing CVD.

| Risk factor | Increased risk |
| --- | :---: |
| Hypertension | x 1.5 |
| Raised glucose | x 1.8 |
| Raised lipids | x 2.3 |
| Tobacco | x 1.6 |
| Hypertension + Glucose | x 2.8 |
| Hypertension + Lipids | x 3.5 |
| Glucose + Lipids | x 4 |
| Hypertension + Glucose + lipids | x 6.2 |
| Tobacco + Lipids | x 6 |
| Tobacco + Hypertension | x 4.5 |
| Tobacco + Lipids + Hypertension | x 16 |

Single risk factors convey a certain level of risk. If a patient has more than one risk factor, which is not uncommon, then they interact and amplify the risk. It is therefore important to consider all a patient's risk factors and attempt to address all the risk factors. However, this should not stop you attempting to modify one if it is not possible for whatever reason to attempt to modify all.

**References:**

- ➢ http://www.ncqa.org/portals/0/Publications/Quality%20Profiles/CHAP6_FI G1.gifh
- ➢ Ebrahim Multiple risk factor interventions for primary prevention of CHD Cochrane Database Syst Rev 2000; (2): CD001561

### 3.3 Which of these Risk Factors do you address in Practice?

You should consider how practically to explore cardiovascular risk with patients.

Take for example the 4 patients shown below.

List which of the risk factors you would consider when seeing these patients:

A 40 year old man with a cough.

A 20 year old man with a headache.

A 39 year old woman seeking maternity care.

A 50 year old woman with chest pain.

Consider them and possibly discuss with a colleague whether you would consider it important to explore cardiovascular risk factors with the patient and if not whether you would consider opportunistically exploring cardiovascular risk factors with the patient. Write down what you personally would do with each patient. It may be of use in future practice.

## Case Vignettes

Now consider 4 case vignettes. Consider the clinical features of each case and determine whether the patient is at high or low risk of CVD. Write down the reason why you have made that assessment.

## Case 1

55 year old woman attends for repeat prescription. Hypertensive for 5 years, no cause found. Irregularly attends doctor and BP control poor. Never smoked. BP 179/98 mm Hg. Urine dip ++ protein. Fundoscopy - AV nipping. Creatinine raised. On Amilodipine 5mgm daily.

## Case 2

30 year old woman with type 1 diabetes since childhood. Well-controlled diabetes HbA1c = 6.0% (non-diabetic <6.0%, diabetic target range 6.5% to 7.5%). Non-smoker. BP 110/70. Lipid profile: Total cholesterol 4.0 mmol/l HDL cholesterol 1.3 mmol/l.

**Consider what if this patient had type 2 diabetes?**

## Case 3

62 year old male baker with type 2 diabetes on Glicazide. Smoker 15 cigarettes/day, overweight, alcohol 56 units/week. BP 138/78 (3/12 ago), 164/72 (1/12 ago), 168/104 (2/52 ago).
Total cholesterol 6.3 mmol/l, HDL 0.9 mmol/l. Fasting glucose 15 mmol/l.

**Case 4**

30 year old male office worker. Non-smoker, alcohol 28 units/week. BP 138/78 (3/12 ago), 164/72 (1/12 ago), 160/90 (2/52 ago). Total cholesterol 5.1 mmol/l, HDL 1.7 mmol/l.

**Reference:**

> ➢ Case studies: Dr Neil Chapman Centre for Circulatory Health Imperial College London

A primary care physician in the UK noted that <u>every</u> consultation with a patient was an opportunity to engage in preventive medicine as well as treating the presenting illness. If all of us physicians do this whenever we can within the constraints of our resources then we can improve the health of our patients.

## What can you do?

Consider, what are the local conditions in the UK in relation to CVD risk and how these may be modified?

Consider how causative factors relate to CVD risk management, the problems you may face in engaging with this type of work and consider any practical solutions to these problems. Write these down for future reference.

## In Summary

In this chapter you have:

- Identified and reinforced your knowledge regarding nine modifiable and four non-modifiable cardiovascular risk factors.

- Reflected on which risk factors, if any, you address in your current medical practices.
- Begun to think about stratifying patients as high risk or low risk based on clinical presentations in case vignettes.
- Begun to consider which individuals might benefit from changing behaviour and lifestyle modification.
- Begun to consider local issues in the UK that might affect your ability to engage in CVD prevention.

# 4. Clinical Risk Assessment for CVD

## Key Points

- The steps involved in clinically assessing patients for CVD.
- The concept of quantifying and communicating cardiovascular risk to patients.

## Objectives

- To describe a logical approach to assessing cardiovascular risk, in the form of history, examination and investigations.
- To feel confident in the use of risk calculating tools such as QRISK2 &/or HeartScore.
- To understand how risk scores influence clinical management and the importance of clear communication of risk to patients.

## 4.1 Why is Clinical Risk Assessment Important?

Despite awareness of CVD as a major health and social problem, many patients at risk remain undiagnosed. Many of those who are diagnosed are undermanaged and show little or no improvement in their levels of risk over time.

A recent comprehensive study in general practice demonstrated the scope for improvement in assessment and treatment for prevention of CVD. Only one third of all patients in the study were receiving optimal treatment.

**Reference:**

> Sheppard Missed opportunities in prevention of CVD in primary care Br J Gen Pract 2014; 64:28-29

### 4.2 What are the Risk Factors for CVD?

In order to consider clinical risk assessment we need to be clear what the risk factors are that we are going to assess?

These risk factors are summarized below:

**Fixed risk factors:** Age, Gender, Ethnicity, Family history.

**Modifiable risk factors:** Smoking, Alcohol, Diet, Weight, Physical activity, Stress, Blood pressure, Lipids, Diabetes.

**Reference:**

> World Heart Federation Fact sheet Cardiovascular disease risk factors 2015

### 4.3 What are the Aims of Cardiovascular Risk Assessment?

- To reduce the incidence of CVD in the community.
- To identify those individuals at risk.
- To improve the quality of life.
- To improve life expectancy.
- To reduce the economic impact of chronic heart disease and stroke.
- Both fixed and modifiable risk factors must be considered. Reducing their effect is a key element of primary healthcare

and one in which all primary care health professionals have a role to play.

**Reference:**

➤ http://cks.nice.org.uk/cvd-risk-assessment-and-management 2014

### 4.4 Who needs a Cardiovascular Risk Assessment?

Here we show you who should have a cardiovascular risk assessment.

- Risk assessment should be routinely offered to all patients known to be at increased risk, that is all people with:
- Hypertension.
- Type 2 Diabetes.
- A strong family history of CVD.
- It should also be offered when the opportunity arises to all adults from age 40-75 years as part of their general primary health care.

**Reference:**

➤ Healthcare Improvement Scotland sign 97 risk estimation and the prevention of cardiovascular disease 2013

### 4.5 Who does not need a Cardiovascular Risk Assessment?

Certain groups of the population do not require risk assessment.

Risk assessment is not required in healthy individuals under 40 years old or people already known to be at high risk (above 20% risk), that is those who:

- Are aged 85 years or more.

- Have established CVD.
- Have a familial hyperlipidaemia.
- Have type 1 diabetes mellitus.
- Have chronic kidney disease.

**Reference:**

➢ NICE Clinical Knowledge summary CVD risk assessment & management 2014

## 4.6 What does Risk Assessment involve?

Imagine you are in the consulting room with a 48 year old male patient and you decide to undertake a cardiovascular risk assessment. What would you actually do?

You apply the basic clinical process of history taking, examination, investigation.

**History:**

Firstly, if not already on file, you would record their age, gender and ethnicity.

Next you discuss their lifestyle history including smoking, alcohol, diet, exercise and stress. Also discuss family history of CVD. Ask about other manifestations, such as erectile dysfunction, intermittent claudication, chest discomfort or dyspnoea on exertion. Enquire about their past medical problems.

**Physical examination:**

- measure height, weight, waist circumference, pulse (rate and rhythm), blood pressure.
- test urine with dip stick test for protein and glucose.
- depending on history and other findings consider further examination of cardiovascular system, for example, assessing heart size, heart sounds, carotid arteries, peripheral pulses, retinal fundi.

**Investigation:**

In light of the above consider the necessity for blood tests for renal function, liver function, lipids, glucose, HbA1c and ECG.

Once all risk factors have been identified, a variety of cardiovascular risk charts or calculators can be used to estimate the total risk of developing CVD over the following 10 years. A total CVD risk of 20% or higher over 10 years is currently defined as high risk.

### 4.6.1 Erectile Dysfunction (ED)

Is common in patients with CVD and confers an additional independent risk assessment factor for future cardiovascular events, usually with a 3-year time period between onset of ED and CVD. In about 25% of cases there is a psychogenic cause. In those with physical causes smoking, obesity, alcohol, hypertension, diabetes, medication, recreational drugs and endocrinological disorders may be factors.

**Reference:**

➢ European Society of Cardiology (2012) European Guidelines on cardiovascular disease prevention in clinical practice (version 2012). European Heart Journal 33(13), 1635-1671.

## 4.7 What is a positive family history?

Most of the factors in this assessment are quite clear but there is sometimes confusion as to what should be considered a positive family history. As CVD is so common nearly everybody has some degree of family history, but in terms of deciding who is at increased risk, a positive family history is generally considered as satisfying one or more of the following criteria:

- Father or brother who developed heart disease or had a stroke before they were aged 55.
- Mother or sister who developed heart disease or had a stroke before they were aged 65.
- Any first degree relative (parent, brother, sister, child) with a serious hereditary lipid disorder, such as familial hyperlipidaemia or familial combined hyperlipidaemia.

**Reference:**

➢ McCusker M Family history of heart disease and cardiovascular disease risk-reducing behaviours. Genet Med. 2004 May-Jun; 6(3):153-8

## 4.8 Cardiovascular Risk Estimation
### Which risk calculators are available?

Once you have completed the clinical risk assessment you need some way of summarising the patient's level of risk in order to record it, communicate it to the patient and make decisions about any measures necessary to reduce their risk.

A variety of cardiovascular risk charts or calculators can be used to estimate the total risk of developing CVD over the following 10 years. A total CVD risk of all cardiovascular events of over 20% during the next 10 years is currently defined as high-risk. Some calculators assess the risk of cardiovascular events, such as myocardial infarct (MI); some assess risk of death from a cardiac event.

There are three main scores which should be mentioned:
JBS2
QRISK2
SCORE and HeartScore (which is available in several languages)

### 4.8.1 JBS2 Cardiovascular Risk Estimation

- Previously recommended by NICE.
- Based on Framingham 1991 10 year risk equations.
- It calculates the risk of cardiovascular events.

JBS2 (The Joint British Societies' guidelines) was developed in the UK for use with all adults aged over 40 with no history of CVD or diabetes who are not already on treatment for blood pressure or lipids and for adults aged under 40 with a family history of premature CVD. It should be used once every 5 years.

The risk factors included in the JBS2 scoring system are:

Age (by decade), Gender, Smoking, Diabetes, Systolic blood pressure, Left ventricular hypertrophy, Ratio of total cholesterol to HDL cholesterol.Recent versions can adjust risk on the basis of central obesity, South Asian ethnic origin and impaired fasting glucose.

# JBS2 Risk Prediction Charts

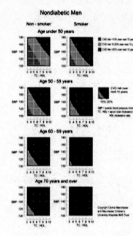
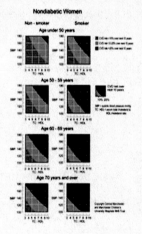

JBS2 is a paper based calculator and uses colour coded risk prediction charts as shown above.

Once you have assessed the patient's risk factors you can choose the appropriate chart and provide a score to estimate their risk of developing CVD within the next 10 years.

**Reference:**
> www.bhsoc.org

## 4.8.2 QRISK2 CVD Risk Calculator

Currently favoured by NICE.

The QRISK2 Score is a risk calculator which can be used on computer, ipad or iphone.

It calculates the risk of cardiovascular events.

It is a development of an earlier QRISK1 Score which was originally developed and validated on large general practice databases in the UK using data from three million patients.

QRISK1 includes the same risk factors as JBS2 i.e. age, gender, smoking, systolic blood pressure and ratio of total cholesterol/HDL but it also includes:

- body mass index.
- family history of CVD.

- social deprivation (Townsend score based on households without a car, overcrowded households, households not owner-occupied, persons unemployed).
- use of antihypertensive treatment.

In addition to the QRISK1 risk factors QRISK2 also includes:

- ethnicity (self-assigned) – Several conditions associated with cardiovascular risk (including diagnosed type 2 diabetes, treated hypertension, rheumatoid arthritis, renal disease, and atrial fibrillation).
- interactions between age and deprivation score, body mass index, systolic blood pressure, family history, smoking status, treated hypertension, diagnosis of type 2 diabetes, and atrial fibrillation.

Age (25-84): [ 64 ]

Sex: ⊙ Male ○ Female

Ethnicity: [ White or not stated ▾ ]

UK postcode: leave blank if unknown

Postcode: [     ]

---

Clinical information

Smoking status: [ non-smoker ▾ ]

Diabetes status: [ none ▾ ]

Angina or heart attack in a 1st degree relative < 60? ☐

Chronic kidney disease (stage 4 or 5)? ☐

Atrial fibrillation? ☐

On blood pressure treatment? ☐

Rheumatoid arthritis? ☐

Leave blank if unknown

Cholesterol/HDL ratio: [     ]

Systolic blood pressure (mmHg): [     ]

Body mass index

Height (cm): [     ]

Weight (kg): [     ]

Calculate risk over [ 10 ▾ ] years. [ Calculate risk ]

**Your results**

Your risk of having a heart attack or stroke within the next 10 years is:

13.5%

In other words, in a crowd of 100 people with the same risk factors as you, 14 are likely to have a heart attack or stroke within the next 10 years.

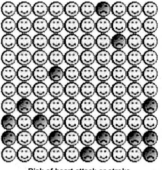

**Risk of heart attack or stroke**

Your score has been calculated using estimated data, as some information was left blank.

Your body mass index was estimated as 27.3 kg/m$^2$.

## How does your 10-year score compare?

Your score

| | |
|---|---|
| Your 10-year QRISK®2 score | 13.5% |
| The score of a healthy person with the same age, sex, and ethnicity* | 12.6% |
| Relative risk** | 1.1 |
| Your QRISK® Healthy Heart Age*** | 66 |

* This is the score of a healthy person of your age, sex and ethnic group, i.e. with no adverse clinical indicators and a cholesterol ratio of 4.0, systolic blood pressure of 125 and BMI of 25.

** Your relative risk is your risk divided by the healthy person's risk.

*** Your QRISK® Healthy Heart Age is the age at which a healthy person of your sex and ethnicity has your 10-year QRISK®2 score.

## Reference:

➢ http://qrisk.org

### 4.8.3 SCORE and HeartScore

**SCORE** (Systematic COronary Risk Evaluation) is a paper-based system similar to JBS2 developed by the European Society of Cardiology (ESC) using data from 12 European cohort studies. It is available in 17 languages.

HeartScore is the interactive version of SCORE. The SCORE risk estimation is based on gender, age, smoking, systolic blood pressure and total cholesterol. It is available in several languages, including Russian.

Note that Score and HeartScore calculators give a score in terms of ten year risk of FATAL CVD.

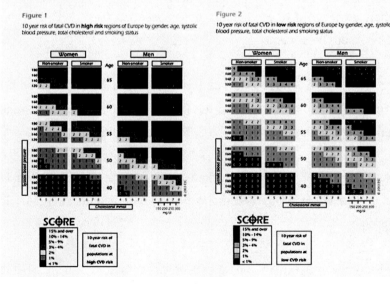

Two versions of the SCORE Chart are available. One is for countries listed by the European Society of Cardiology as having low risk for CVD and the other for countries considered as having high risk (which includes Russia).

Again take the example of our 48 year old male smoker and give him a cholesterol of 7.0 and a systolic blood pressure of 160.

So using the chart:
1. find the cell nearest to the patient's age, cholesterol and BP values;
2. check the qualifiers;
3. establish the total 10 year risk for fatal CVD.

Using the chart for risk assessment gives a lower estimate of risk than using QRISK as SCORE only assesses fatal CVD and the QRISK all CVD events.

## Risk estimation using SCORE: Qualifiers

The charts should be used in the light of the clinician's knowledge and judgement, especially with regard to local conditions.

As with all risk estimation systems, risk will be overestimated in countries with a falling CVD mortality rate, and underestimated if it is rising.

At any given age, risk appears lower for women than men. This is misleading since, ultimately, more women than men die from CVD.

Inspection of the charts shows that their risk is merely deferred by 10 years.

**Risk may be higher than indicated in the chart in:**

- Sedentary or obese subjects, especially those with central obesity.
- Those with a strong family history of premature CVD.
- The socially deprived.
- Diabetics. Risk may be 5 fold higher in women with diabetes and 3 fold higher in men with diabetes compared to those without diabetes.
- Those with low HDL cholesterol or high triglycerides.
- Asymptomatic subjects with evidence of pre-clinical atherosclerosis, for example a reduced ankle-brachial index or on imaging such as carotid ultrasonography or CT scanning.

## HeartScore

HeartScore is the interactive on-line version of SCORE.

Like SCORE it estimates 10 year risk of fatal cardiovascular events based on:

Gender, Age, Smoking, systolic blood pressure, total cholesterol. Recently HDL, BMI and 'risk age' function have been included.

*(The 'risk age' function determines the theoretical age of a person exposed to the same range and level of risk factors – this will help patients quickly understand their exposure to overall CVD risk).*

However because it has interactive functionality HeartScore also provides:

Patient history and progress management, Patient list management, Graphical display of absolute CVD risk, Graphical display of risk factors contribution to total risk, Links to European guidelines on CVD Prevention in clinical practice, Printable patient advice. Access is free for health professionals.

**Reference:**

> http://www.heartscore.org/Pages/welcome.aspx

### What does the HeartScore result mean?

In SCORE and HeartScore patients are given a ten year percentage risk of a FATAL cardiovascular event. This is different from other risk assessment tools which are based on fatal and non-fatal events. This is somewhat controversial but the argument is that in terms of risk research death is clearly a defined and measurable outcome, whereas non-fatal events such as angina, MI, stroke are less strictly defined and measured.

So in SCORE and HeartScore a result of 30% means that the patient has a 30% chance of dying from CVD within the next 10 years.

Patients scoring 5% or less are regarded as low risk and should be offered advice to maintain their low-risk status.

Those with a risk of 5-10% qualify for intensive life-style modification advice, and may benefit from drug treatment.

In general for those at risk levels of 10% or more drug treatment is usually required in addition to life-style modification.

Those with a risk of 20% or greater require life-style modification and drug treatment including prophylactic statins.

There is discussion, at the present time, whether a 10% level of risk of **all** cardiovascular events should be the level at which life-style changes and prophylactic use of statins should be routinely introduced.

In people over 60 these thresholds should be interpreted more leniently, because their age-specific risk (that is the risk of having a fatal cardiovascular event based on age alone) is >10%, even when other cardiovascular risk factor levels are 'normal'.

Note that the relative risk chart in black and white at the bottom of the SCORE chart may be helpful in identifying and counseling in young people, even if absolute risk levels are low. This will be discussed again when we explain absolute and relative risk in detail.

**Reference:**
- European Heart Journal, 2003, 24; 987-1003

### 4.9 Absolute and Relative Risk

### What are absolute and relative risks?

**Absolute risk** of a disease is your risk of developing the disease over a given time period. We all have absolute risks of developing various diseases such as heart disease, cancer, stroke etc.

The same absolute risk can be expressed in different ways. For example, say you have a 1 in 10 risk of developing a certain disease in your life. This can also be said to be a 10% risk, or a 0.1 risk - depending whether you use percentages or decimals.

**Relative risk** is used to compare the risk in two different groups of people. For example smokers and non-smokers or diabetics and non-diabetics.

An example may illustrate this better:
If we know from research that 6 in 100 SMOKERS (6%) will develop condition X but only 4 in 100 NON-SMOKERS (4%) will develop condition X.

The **ABSOLUTE RISK** (AR) of developing condition X is 6 in 100 for smokers and 4 in 100 for non-smokers.

In other words, comparing smokers with non-smokers, the risk of developing Condition X is 50% greater relative to smokers (6 - 4 / 4 x 100).
Smokers therefore have a **RELATIVE RISK** of 50%.

Notice that a 50% difference sounds more impressive than the Absolute Risk Reduction (ARR) which is 2% (4%-2%) although both these numbers describe the same difference.

**Reference:**
 ➢ Cancer Research UK Science blog Absolute versus relative risk – making sense of media stories 2013

### 4.9.1 Relative Risk Assessment

The relative risk chart included in HeartScore may be used to show younger people at low absolute risk that, relative to others in their age group, their risk may be many times higher than expected. This may help motivate changes in lifestyle and help decisions around when to start medication.

A problem in assessing risk in younger people (below age 50) is that a low absolute risk may conceal a very high relative or lifetime risk.

Note that this chart shows RELATIVE not absolute risk. The risks are RELATIVE to 1 in the bottom left box. Thus a person in the top right hand box has a risk that is 12 times higher than a person in the bottom left.

**Reference:**
 ➢ http://www.heartscore.org/Pages/background.aspx

### 4.9.2 Risk Age Assessment

HeartScore also now includes a 'risk age' function that determines the theoretical age of a person exposed to the same range and level of risk factors. For example you can show a 40 year old male smoker that his risk factor although relatively low at 3% is the same as that of a 60 year old man who doesn't smoke. This can help patients quickly understand their exposure to overall CVD risk.

**Reference:**

> ➢ http://www.ncbi.nlm.nih.gov/pubmed/22626902

### 4.10 Proposed Alternative Risk Calculators

None of the existing risk calculators are perfect. They all either under- or overestimate risks. Numerous researchers and clinicians are seeking more specific risk markers. A recent proposal is shown here.

**Pooled Cohort CVD Risk Equations** are based on data easily available to primary care advisers which could be implemented in clinical practice. They do not use the Framingham algorithm, but are derived from community based cohorts and estimate 10 year risk of developing first CVD events, fatal or non-fatal MI and fatal or non-fatal stroke. They thus take into account ethnic diversity.

**References:**

> ➢ ACC/AHA Guideline on the Assessment of CV risk: A report of the American College of Cardiology & American Heart Association Task Force on Practice Guidelines 2013

> Cooney Value & Limitations of existing Scores for Assessment of Cardiovascular Risk Jour Am Coll Card Vol 54, Issue 14 2009 1209-1227

## 4.11 Novel Markers for Risk

We show below some possible alternatives markers of cardiac risk. None have yet been considered suitable for routine use in clinical risk assessment in the general population.

Coronary artery calcium (CAC)

C reactive protein (CRP)

Fibrinogen

Lipoproteins

Homocysteine

NT ProBPN

Plasma Retinol

Genetic marker

Carotid intima-media thickness (assessed by Ultra Sound Scan or MRI)

Ankle brachial index

**References:**

> Qureshi Introducing genetic testing for CVD in primary care Br J Gen Pract 2014; 64:234-235

> Comparison of Novel Risk Markers for Improvement in Cardiovascular Risk Assessment in Intermediate-Risk Individuals JAMA. 2012; 308(8):788-795

## 4.12 Informing Patients about their Health Risks

A major challenge in preventive medicine is how to inform patients about their health risks and the benefits of possible treatment options in a way they will understand, remember and comply with.

**Reference:**
  ➢ Health affairs 30, no. 4 (2011): the people-to-people health foundation, inc

## 4.13 Health Literacy

Health literacy is an individual's ability to read, understand and use healthcare information to make decisions and follow instructions for treatment.

This is a relatively new area of research but evidence in the UK and USA shows surprisingly low levels of health literacy and numeracy.

Presenting relative as opposed to absolute risk is a useful option for discussing CVD risk especially with younger adults.

**Reference:**
  ➢ WHO. Background Note: Regional Preparatory Meeting on Promoting Health Literacy [Internet]. UN ECOSOC, 2009

## 4.14 Presenting Risk to Patients

Patients need to know:
- What is my risk of developing CVD?
- What can I do to reduce the risk?
- How effective will this be?

## How best to present risk?

- Keep it clear and simple.
- Use graphs and pictures.
- Present in context of everyday things.
- Give appropriate perspective.

*"The bad news is your risk has doubled - the good news is it has gone from one in a million to two in a million".*

Risk can be communicated by:

- **words** such as *"your risk is high"* or *"this is not good for your health"*).
- **numbers** - absolute percentages, relative percentages, natural frequencies.
- **visual formats** - pictures, graphs, bar charts, pie charts.
- **or by a combination of these methods.**

Although there is no clear evidence as to which format is the best for communicating risk most effectively, recent research suggests that the use of natural frequencies, graphical formats (e.g. bar charts), and combinations of these are more effective than percentages or a purely verbal communication of risk.

The clinician must also take into account the fact that patients understanding of and ability to comply with advice will be influenced by such factors as age, education, literacy, numeracy, cultural and socioeconomic background.

Growing evidence suggests that involving patients in decision-making has positive effects in terms of patient satisfaction, compliance, and even health outcomes. Patients are increasingly seeking more active participation in healthcare decisions and wanting a shift towards a meaningful dialogue with their doctors.

**Reference:**

> Communicating Risk BMJ 2012; 344:e3996

## 4.15 Barriers to Risk Assessment

- Oversimplification.
- Poor patient understanding.
- Lack of time.
- Possible overestimation of risk.
- Possible misuse of medical therapy.
- Higher health costs.

We have discussed why risk assessment is important and some of the tools available to help us. We have also shown how these can be used in the clinic setting.

It is understood however that that there are a number of barriers to implementing the existing risk assessments in clinical practice.

A survey among general practitioners and internists working in clinical practice in two Swiss regions revealed that 74% rarely or never used CVD prediction charts due to fears of oversimplification of risk assessment and belief that the numerical information resulting from prediction rules is frequently unhelpful for clinical decision-making.

We also know that patients may have a limited understanding of risk tables and how risk relates to disease development.

The length of routine patient consultations often provides little time for discussion and risk assessment is yet another item to take up limited time.

There are also concerns about overestimating risk in national populations, which may lead to overuse of medical therapy. Results of a Norwegian study suggest that using the SCORE assessment routinely would double the number of individuals who need drugs for primary prevention of CVD and thus possibly increase numbers developing serious side effects from the medication. Increasing numbers of patients receiving medications may result in higher healthcare costs.

Health economists however argue that by reducing CVD risk there should be long term savings in healthcare costs by reducing overall CVD levels in the community.

**Reference:**

➤ Crosson Physicians' perceptions of barriers to CVD risk factor control among patients with diabetes: (TRIAD) study. J Am Board Fam Med. 2010 Mar-Apr; 23(2):171-8

## In Summary

In this chapter we have discussed the steps involved in clinically assessing patients for CVD, and the concept of quantifying and communicating cardiovascular risk.

You should now be able to:
- Describe a logical approach to assessing cardiovascular risk, in the form of history, examination, and investigations.
- Feel confident in the use of risk calculating tools such as HeartScore and/or QRISK2.
- Understand how risk scores influence clinical management and the importance of clear communication with patients.

Evidence shows, that by incorporating these simple checks into the routine of primary health care you can over time make a real difference in terms of reducing CVD morbidity and mortality.

### Risk assessment role play

Now organise a risk assessment role play with your colleagues. One of you, male or female, plays the part of the doctor and the other is the patient.

### Case Vignette

55 year old man. Smokes 30 cigarettes a day. Not diabetic. Total cholesterol 5.9 mmol/l. HDL cholesterol 1.3 mmol/l. Systolic BP 125mm Hg.

What advice would you give him and how would you treat him?

## Lifestyle Modifications

## 5. Smoking

### Key Points

- Globally smoking is the leading preventable cause of disease and death.
- Tobacco is probably the single most important modifiable risk factor for CVD.
- Most smokers say that they would like to quit.
- Cessation advice can help them to stop smoking.
- Primary Care Practitioners are in a unique position to encourage patients to stop smoking.

In this chapter we look at smoking. We will consider how smoking affects both cardiovascular and general health, the prevalence of smoking in the UK and the effects on mortality.

We will then consider in depth how you as GPs/Healthcare professionals can help your patients to quit the habit, using a 'best practice' formula for brief interventions.

The aims of the chapter are to be able to promote the cardiovascular health of your patients by educating them about smoking.

The objectives are as follows:

- To revise the risks of developing CVD from smoking.
- To be able to assess a patient's dependence and willingness to quit smoking.

- To learn about smoking cessation adjuncts.
- To encourage your patients to change their behaviour and modify their lifestyle.

### 5.1 Smoking - Key Facts

- Globally smoking is the leading preventable cause of disease and death. It kills six million people worldwide annually. Every 6.5 seconds someone dies from tobacco use. As well as causing heart disease, chronic obstructive pulmonary disease (COPD) and lung cancer, smoking has the ability to harm every organ of the body.
- People who start smoking in their teens and continue for two decades or more will die 20 to 25 years earlier than those who have never smoked.
- A female smoker has a greater risk of developing CVD than a male smoker.
- Passive smoking (secondhand smoking) also leads to increased risk of CVD.

But, smoking is a modifiable behaviour and stopping smoking brings immediate and long term health benefits. Most smokers say that they would like to quit, but most don't know how to go about it and lack the motivation and knowledge to succeed. Cessation advice can help and Primary Care doctors are in a unique position to encourage their patients to stop smoking. Quit lines, pharmacological therapies and behaviour therapies are effective interventions.

**Reference:**

➢ http://www.ash.org.uk/files/documents/ASH_113.pdf

## 5.2 Nicotine Dependence

- Genetic factors may influence the response of specific receptors in the brain to high doses of nicotine.
- Home and peer influence. Children with family and friends who smoke are more likely to smoke.
- Smoking on television, films and on the stage encourages smoking.
- The younger you start smoking the greater the chance of becoming a heavy smoker.
- Sufferers from depression, schizophrenia and PTSD are more likely to smoke.
- Those who drink alcohol and illegal drug users are more likely to smoke.

### 5.2.1 Harmful Effects of Nicotine

Causes mood alterations by acting as a stimulant or relaxant. Increases heart rate, raises blood pressure, vaso-constricts and aggravates diabetes.

**Reference:**

➢ Psychology today

https://www.psychologytoday.com/conditions/nicotine 2014

## 5.3 Tobacco Smoking

- Mortality from CVD increases with age and increasing amounts of tobacco smoked. A person's risk increases if they started smoking as a child.

- The risk increases if the smoker is a woman. If a woman smokes 3 to 5 cigarettes a day, she doubles her risk of heart attack. A man would have to smoke 6 to 9 cigarettes a day to double his risk.

- There are certain people who are more susceptible to the effects of smoking. About 25% of the population have a gene that increases their risk of developing coronary heart disease by up to four times.

- We should not forget that those people exposed to tobacco smoke in the work place or home are also at increased risk due to their exposure (passive or secondhand smoking).

- The good news is that if a person stops smoking their risk of CVD decreases to almost the same as a non-smoker over time and that this happens however long the person has smoked.

**PEOPLE SHOULD ALWAYS BE ENCOURAGED TO STOP SMOKING.**

**Reference:**

➢ How Tobacco Smoke Causes Disease: The Biology and Behavioral Basis for Smoking-Attributable Disease: A Report of the Surgeon General NCBI Centers for Disease Control & Prevention (US) 2010

## 5.4 Passive Smoking

Passive smoking occurs on breathing in other people's smoke. This can increase the risk of CVD and cancer, and can cause other health problems, including stroke and breathing problems. The level of mortality from cardio-vascular diseases in families where one member is a smoker is 20% higher than in non-smoking families. In families who use tobacco, a child is twice as likely to smoke as in a family which doesn't. In addition, children of parents who smoke have higher rates of respiratory and middle ear infections, asthma and meningococcal infections.

**Reference:**

➢ Lightwood Declines in acute MI after smoke free laws and individual risk attributed to secondhand smoke Circulation 2009; 120:1373-1379

## 5.5 Smoking during Pregnancy

**Risks to mother:** Placental abruption, placenta praevia, premature rupture of membranes, spontaneous abortion, ectopic pregnancy.

**Risks to foetus, infants, children:** Stunted gestational development, stillbirth, sudden infant death syndrome, reduced lung function and impaired lung development, asthma and bronchitis exacerbations, acute lower respiratory infections (bronchitis and pneumonia), respiratory irritation (cough, phlegm wheeze), childhood cancers, orofacial cleft, possible increased risk of allergic conditions, possible increased risk learning difficulties and attention-deficit/hyperactivity disorder (ADHD).

## 5.6 How Tobacco harms you

Most people know that tobacco is harmful, but few even among health professionals understand just how dangerous it is.

Smoking is one of the biggest risk factors for developing CVD. It is estimated that smoking-related CVD kills more than 600,000 people each year in developed countries. Smoking makes the heart beat faster, increases the risk of hypertension, produces carbon monoxide which damages the endothelium of blood vessels and eventually causes heart attacks and strokes.

- Smokers have 10 times the risk of ischaemic heart disease (IHD) compared with non-smokers, and are four times more likely than non-smokers to die from heart disease.
- In addition to the CVD risk smoking increases the risk of developing many cancers.
- Smokers are 20 times more likely to develop lung cancer than non-smokers. The longer one smokes, the greater the risk of developing other cancers: nasal and para-nasal, oral, naso-pharyngeal, oro- and hypo-pharyngeal, laryngeal, oesophageal, stomach, pancreas, kidney, bladder, breast.
- Smoking also causes emphysema and Chronic Obstructive Pulmonary Disease (COPD).
- Other conditions associated with smoking are stomach ulcers, osteoporosis, gum disease and tooth decay, hearing loss, psoriasis, cataracts and macular degeneration and dementia.

- In addition smoking is associated with gender specific conditions. Impotence, infertility and deformed sperm in men, and cervical cancer, fertility problems, and lower oestrogen levels in women. Women who are on oral contraceptives and smoke have a 20% increased risk of stroke and subarachnoid haemorrhage.
- Smoking during pregnancy increases the risk of spontaneous abortion, low weight babies, stillbirths, placental abnormalities and has an adverse impact on development of the foetus including congenital heart disease.

And if you are not already convinced. Smoking also increases risk of complications of diabetes, slows down the healing of wounds, and causes wrinkles.

**References:**

➢ The Tobacco Atlas 5th edition Chapter 3 Health consequences 18-19
➢ Edwards The problem of tobacco smoking BMJ 2004; 328:217-219

## 5.7 The Benefits of Quitting

Quitting smoking brings with it immediate and long-term sustained benefits.

20 minutes    Blood pressure and heart rate return to normal.

8 hours    Nicotine and carbon monoxide levels in blood decrease by 50%, oxygen levels return to normal.

| | |
|---|---|
| 24 hours | Carbon monoxide eliminated from body. Lungs start to clear out mucus and other debris. |
| 48 hours | There is no nicotine in the body. Ability to taste and smell are greatly improved. |
| 2-12 weeks | Circulation will be improving. |
| 3-9 months | Coughs, wheezing and breathing problems improve as lung function increases by up to 10%. |
| 1 year | Risk of heart attack falls to about half that of a smoker. |
| 10 years | Risk of lung cancer falls to about half that of a smoker. Risk of heart attack falls to the same as someone who has never smoked. |

**Reference:**

➤ The benefits of stopping smoking Patient.co.uk
http://patient.info/health/the-benefits-of-stopping-smoking 2015

## 5.8 Cigarette Smoking in the UK

- Smoking is responsible for one third of all CVD deaths in Western populations.
- In 1984 in the UK 82% men and 41% women smoked. By 2010 this had fallen to 21% men and 20% women. In 2013 22.6% males and 17.6% females were smoking.
- However in the UK, 10 Million adults still smoke. Smokers average 12.7 cigarettes a day.
- 25% males aged 25-34 years smoke, but only 11% males aged over 60 years smoke. Figures for females are respectively 29% and 13%.
- In 2011 1.5 million hospital admissions were for smoking-related illnesses. 79,000 deaths in over 35s were caused by

smoking-related diseases (18% of all deaths in that age group). 100,000 deaths annually are due to smoking-related diseases.

- In 2013 12% of professionals and 29% of manual workers smoked.
- Regionally smoking rates vary from 22.3% in NE England to 17.2% in SE England.
- UK households spent £18.3 million on tobacco in 2011.
- In 2014-2015 UK tax revenue from tobacco was £9.5 billion. Government expenditure in 2012-2013 on smoking prevention measures was £87 million plus £58 million on anti-smoking medication.

**References:**

➢ Office for National Statistics Statistical Bulletin Adult Smoking Habits in Great Britain, 2013
➢ NHS Health & Social Care Information Centre 2012 Statistics on smoking England 2014
  http://www.hscic.gov.uk/pubs/smoking15
➢ ASH Fact sheet on Smoking statistics - illness & death 2015

## 5.8.1 Tobacco and CVD in Scotland

- In 2010 26% men and 25% women smoked in Scotland.
- Down from 46% in 1970. By 2013 this had fallen further to 23% of total Scottish population.
- In 2009 there were 13,000 deaths from smoking-related illness in Scotland.

- Tobacco smoking prevalence is higher in Scotland than in England and Wales.
- Prevalence is twice as high in routine and manual occupations compared with managerial and professional.
- Four in ten people in Scotland's most deprived areas smoke.
- Almost one third of deaths in those areas are due to smoking, compared with 15% in affluent areas.
- Since introduction in Scotland in 2006 of smoke-free public places hospital admissions for acute coronary syndrome have fallen by 17% and second hand smoking exposure by 39%.

**References:**

➢ British Heart Foundation CHD Statistics in Scotland 2012
➢ ASH Scotland report 2011 & 2012
➢ Scottish Public Health Observatory report 2012

## 5.9 Tobacco Control Measures in the UK

- Sales are not permitted to minors under the age of 18 years.
- Smoking is not permitted under the age of 16 years.
- Advertising, promotion and sponsorship are not permitted.
- Health warnings are compulsory on cigarette packs.
- Smoking bans are mandatory in workplaces and public places since 2007.
- High taxation levels equating to 57% of cost.
- Anti-smoking campaigns.
- Measures to limit tobacco smuggling.

- With the aim of reducing adult smoking levels by 2015 from 21% to 18.5% of the population (15 year olds from 15% to 12% and pregnant women from 14% to 11%), the following proposals were made in 2011 by the government:
- Non-display of tobacco in large shops from 2012 and small shops from 2015. Plain packaging of cigarettes is due to commence in 2016.

**Reference:**

➤ Healthy living, healthy people. A tobacco control plan for England 2011 to 2015

### 5.10 Why do People Smoke?

Arguably the most important cause of smoking is the influence of tobacco advertising and promotion.

Culturally acceptable.

To cope with stress.

Use smoking as a support for when things go wrong.

Enjoy smoking with others as a shared activity.

Use smoking to start conversations and meet new people.

Smoke to make themselves look more confident and in control.

Think that cigarettes help them to keep their weight down.

Have a cigarette when they're feeling bored or lonely.

Smoke when they need a break or a moment to themselves.

Peer example and pressures.

**Reference:**

➤ http://healthliteracy.worlded.org/docs/tobacco/Unit3/1why_people_smoke.html

## 5.11 Why Stopping Smoking may be difficult

You may well ask, *If smoking is known to be bad for health, and quitting can bring such benefits then why don't more people quit?*

Nicotine is the component of cigarette smoke responsible for the addictive properties of cigarette smoking. In both the central and peripheral nervous systems, nicotine acts as an agonist at ganglionic cholinergic receptors and causes the release of neurotransmitters including dopamine, noradrenaline, acetylcholine and serotonin.

Stopping smoking can lead to withdrawal and craving. These and other symptoms can cause smokers to relapse.

In addition to physiological dependence there is often a strong psychological dependence. Tobacco smoking is a complex acquired behaviour and strongly embedded habit. The smoker needs to learn skills that will help control his/her behaviour.

Several of the effects of nicotine are perceived by smokers as being desirable and may motivate the continuation of smoking. For example, beliefs that smoking increases positive mood, improves memory, reduces tension and stress and helps relaxation.

People may be also be reluctant to quit because of the prospect of losing a favourite pastime, environmental factors that perpetuate smoking, or fear of gaining weight.

**Reference:**

> ➢ Understanding motivation might be the key to quitting smoking. All About Addiction 2012

## 5.12 Stopping smoking as a process

Changing behaviour is a complex process that can require many attempts before success is achieved. People move from having no motivation to change their behaviour to the eventual internalization of healthy behaviour. Several models map the changes which determine behaviour and behaviour change. For example the Stages of Change model described by Prochaska and Di Clemente, which broadly describes the process of changing through no contemplation of quitting to thinking about quitting, to preparing and to action (see chapter 2).

People do not always move through the stages in a linear fashion. People may either move forward or backward through different stages of change as their attitudes toward the behaviour alter. At each consultation, it is useful to identify the smoker's interest in quitting at that point in time and targeting appropriate intervention accordingly. Moving a smoker from one stage to a stage closer to quitting is a 'successful' management step.

**Not interested in changing:** not currently considering change or have any intention to change behaviour in the near future. They may be unaware a problem exists.
Patient requires information and education to change attitudes.

**Thinking about change:** aware that a problem exists and seriously thinking about overcoming it but not yet made a commitment to take action. Still not sure if the long-term benefits outweigh the short-term costs.

Patient needs to weigh the pros and cons of changing.

**Preparing to change:** made a commitment to start usually involving developing strategies and identifying resources to help.

You must give advice and encouragement.

**Making changes:** involves the most time and energy and is often the period of the greatest risk for relapse.

Patient requires help and support.

**Maintaining change:** attempt to maintain the new behaviour and resist the temptation to relapse.

You need to give continued support.

**Relapse:** It is normal to cycle through the stages more than once, as relapse is inherent.

While relapse can be discouraging, it's important to consider what triggered a relapse, and to restart the process again at the preparation, action or maintenance stage.

**Reference:**

➢ Velicer Applications of the Transtheoretical Model: Smoking cessation & stress management Homeostasis; 38:216-233

### 5.12.1 What Primary Care Doctors can do to help

Primary Care Practitioners are in a unique position to encourage patients to stop smoking. The Primary Care practitioner clearly has a legitimate role in asking all patients whether they smoke or not. The question is not an invasion of the patient's life style choices, but one of concern about the patient's health status.

Additionally, smoking can increase the risk of adverse outcomes when combined with commonly prescribed medications such as the oral contraceptive pill and hormone replacement therapies, so this interaction needs to be considered by the practitioner.

An assessment of the individual's commitment to quit should be undertaken. Then brief interventions should be initiated.

Brief interventions can increase cessation rates significantly and can be used with all populations including adolescents, pregnant women, older smokers, smokers with medical co-morbidities, smokers with mental illness, and racial and ethnic minorities, and can be applied to all current tobacco users, not just those willing to make a quit attempt. They can also enhance motivation to quit in those not yet ready.

The content of the intervention will depend on a number of factors, including the individual's willingness to quit, how acceptable they find the intervention on offer and the previous ways they have tried to quit. It will involve opportunistic advice, discussion, negotiation or encouragement and referral for more intensive treatment, where appropriate.

The goal is to ensure that every patient who uses tobacco is identified and offered at least a brief intervention at each clinical visit.

Further measures such as Pharmacotherapy and behavioural support, Self-help material and Referral for more intensive support should be offered when appropriate.

### 5.12.2 Best Practice Brief Intervention: The 5As

Let us show you a helpful outline for managing patients who are smokers by brief interventions. The best practice brief intervention is the 5As model. This 'best practice' model is recommended in the US guidelines and comprises five major steps in providing a brief intervention in the primary care setting.

The steps are: (1) **Ask** the patient if he or she uses tobacco, (2) **Advise** him or her to quit, (3) **Assess** willingness to make a quit attempt, (4) **Assist** those who are willing to make a quit attempt, and (5) **Arrange** for follow-up contact to continue support and prevent relapse.

**Reference:**

> ➢ Fiore MC et al. A Clinical Practice Guideline for Treating Tobacco Use and Dependence: 2008 update. A US Public Health Service report. American J of Preventative Medicine, 2008, 35, 158-176

**ASK:** Systematically identify all tobacco users at every consultation. The first step is to ask all patients about their smoking and take a smoking history.

As part of your routine health assessment with all your patients, you should identify your patients' smoking status and document status. At subsequent consultations check the current smoking status of those who have previously quit. At this stage you can also measure their dependence and past quit attempts.

A useful tool for measuring the level of nicotine dependence is the...

### 5.12.3 Fagerström Test for Nicotine Dependence (FTND)

1. How soon after you wake up do you smoke your first cigarette?

| | |
|---|---|
| Within 5 minutes | 3 |
| 6-30 minutes | 2 |
| More than 30 minutes | 0 |

2. Do you find it difficult to stop smoking in no-smoking areas?

| | |
|---|---|
| No | 0 |
| Yes | 1 |

3. Which cigarette would you hate most to give up?

| | |
|---|---|
| The first of the morning | 1 |
| Other | 0 |

4. How many cigarettes a day do you usually smoke?

| | |
|---|---|
| 10 or less | 0 |
| 11 to 20 | 1 |
| 21 to 30 | 2 |
| 31 or more | 3 |

5. Do you smoke more frequently in the first hours after waking than during the rest of the day?

No                          0

Yes                         1

6. Do you smoke if you are so ill that you are in bed most of the day?

No                          0

Yes                         1

The FTND is a validated questionnaire.

In scoring the FTND items are summed to yield a total score of 0-10, and dependence can be scored as follows:

| 0-2 | Very low | 5 | Moderate |
| 3-4 | Low | 6-7 | High |
| | | 8-10 | Very high |

- Ask, *What is the longest time you managed to quit? What helped you at that time?* It is also helpful to know what caused them to relapse. *Why did you fail in your previous attempts?*
- Even if your patient doesn't currently smoke; if they are an ex-smoker then their health can be adversely affected. It is valuable to establish how many a day they smoked, for how long, and when they stopped smoking.
- Also enquire about previous quit attempts (both number and length) and previous use of pharmacotherapy.

**Reference:**

➤ Heatherton TF, Kozlowski LT, Frecker RC, & Fagerström KO. The Fagerström Test for Nicotine Dependence: A revision of the Fagerström Tolerance Questionnaire. Brit J Addict. 1991; 86: 1119-1127

**ADVICE:** Strongly urge all tobacco users to quit.

The next step is to advise all patients who smoke to quit.

The advice should be brief, non-judgmental and should be:

Clear:

*It is important that you quit smoking now and I can help you.*
*I am concerned about your health and feel quitting smoking could be the best thing for your health now. How do you feel about this?*

Strong:

*As your doctor I need you to know that quitting smoking is the most important thing you can do to protect your current and future health. How do you feel about this?*

Personalised and tailored to the individual:

This may involve a discussion of cardiac, vascular and pulmonary symptoms and diseases, or it may involve feedback in regard to results of lung function tests and effects of passive smoking on family members.

*Cutting down while you are ill is not enough.*

*Occasional or light smoking is still dangerous.*

*Continuing to smoke makes your asthma worse and quitting may dramatically improve your health.*

*Quitting smoking may reduce the number of ear infections your child has.*

Provide your patient with accurate information about the consequences of smoking and smoking cessation in a way that maximises motivation to quit or stay quit. Check that the patient understands the risks and benefits, and encourage them to believe that they can succeed.

Information about pharmacological therapies that can support a quit attempt should be provided.

**ASSESS:** Determine willingness to make a quit attempt.

It is important that you tailor your approach to smokers depending on the stage they are at, and this involves assessing the patient's willingness and readiness to make a quit attempt.

Ask, *Are you willing to give quitting a try?*

### 5.12.4 Motivation to Stop Smoking

These questions can be used to assess how much the smoker wants to quit.

1. How important is it to you to give up smoking altogether?

Desperately important

Very important

Quite important

Not all that important

2. How determined are you to give up smoking at this attempt?

Extremely determined

Very determined

Quite determined

Not all that determined

3. Why do you want to give up smoking?

My health is suffering

Worried about future health

It costs too much

Pressure from other people

For my family's health

4. How high would you rate your chances of giving up smoking for good?

Extremely high

Very high

Quite high

Not very high

Low

Very low

**Reference:**

> ➤ Motivation to stop smoking NHS Centre for Smoking Cessation & Training
>
> http://www.ncsct.co.uk/publication_motivation-to-stop-smoking.php

**ASSIST:** Aid the patient in quitting.

If your patient is willing to make a quit attempt at this time, congratulate them on making this decision and help them to develop a quit plan.

- Set a quit date. Ideally, the quit date should be within 2 weeks.
- Identify his/her reasons for wanting to quit.
- Check their expectations of quitting.
- *What could get in your way?*
- *What can you do to help yourself?*
- Encourage the patient to plan ahead to avoid triggers of relapse:
- Anticipate and discuss triggers or challenges in the upcoming attempt and how the patient will successfully overcome them (for example make changes in habitual daily routine, remove tobacco products from the home and environment, make your home smoke-free, try to avoid stressful situations).
- Determine high risk situations for relapsing by asking: *Which cigarette would be hardest to give up? In what situations are you most likely to smoke?*
- Encourage the patient to limit alcohol intake since alcohol is associated with relapse.
- Enlist family support and social support.

- Encourage the patient to tell family, friends and co-workers about quitting and have the patient request their understanding and support.
- Enhance motivation
- Remind patients of the risks and benefits and emphasise that it is never too late to quit.
- Assess confidence to quit by asking patient to self-rate on a scale of 1–10. (10 equates to people who think they can/are more likely to quit than those who don't).
- Boost self-confidence throughout.
- Many patients have successfully stopped smoking. *I believe that you will also be able to do it.*
- Offer printed material support (booklets and brochures).
- Offer the patient questionnaires to complete at home to identify reasons for quitting, and anticipate danger zones.
- Discuss withdrawal symptoms and give practical advice about coping with withdrawal symptoms.
- Describe pharmacological therapies that can support a quit attempt.

**Reference:**
➢ ASH Fact Sheet 7 Stopping smoking: the benefits and aids to quitting 2014


**5.13 Symptoms of Withdrawal and its Management**

Nicotine is an addictive and fast acting drug. When a smoker inhales, nicotine gets into their bloodstream, reaching their brain 10 seconds later. Cessation of the drug can induce withdrawal symptoms in some smokers.

Withdrawal symptoms typically develop after 90 to 120 minutes, reaching a maximum in 24 to 48 hours. Withdrawal symptoms typically last 10–14 days but can last up to 28 days, and in rare cases may persist for some months. These symptoms can include:

- Craving and urges to smoke. Each one lasts a short time, but may be strong. Over time, cravings will happen less often.
- Negative mood and feelings of irritability, depression or anxiety.
- Difficulty concentrating.
- Coughing – this occurs as the cilia in the lung begin to function again.
- Changed sleeping patterns or unusual dreams. However, many people find they sleep better.
- Increase in appetite and possible weight gain. Not everyone gains weight but on average, the weight gain is 3-4 kg.
- Occasional headaches.
- Gastrointestinal problems including constipation, diarrhoea and/or nausea.

Not all smokers will experience withdrawal symptoms, but medication (see 5.14) can help to reduce cravings and withdrawal symptoms.

**Reference:**

> How to handle withdrawal symptoms and triggers when you decide to quit smoking National Cancer Institute Home About Cancer / Causes and Prevention/ Risk Factors/ Tobacco 2010

## 5.14 Pharmacological Interventions

Medication should be offered to all nicotine dependent smokers, except where contraindicated. However, it is not usually recommended for those who smoke less than 10 cigarettes a day *Medication is not a magic cure – but it will help.*

**Nicotine Release Therapy (NRT)** products release a low dosage of nicotine over a sustained period and therefore help reduce nicotine cravings and withdrawal symptoms without the harmful elements of cigarettes.

Using NRT can nearly double the success rate of quitting.

NRT in any form should be used as an adjunct for not longer than 8 to 12 weeks.

Efficiency increases when combined with counselling and social support.

There are a number of different NRT products available that differ in nominal dose and the method and speed of delivery of nicotine.

**Nicotine patches** work by giving a constant supply of nicotine. Available in 16 and 24-hour patches. The 16-hour patch is ideal for most regular smokers. A patch is usually the first choice of NRT as it is the easiest to administer. It can be combined with an intermittent form of NRT if necessary.

**Nicotine gum** gives nicotine on demand. Nicotine is absorbed through the lining of the mouth.

**Microtab** is a small tablet containing nicotine that dissolves under the tongue.

There is also a **nicotine lozenge** which you suck slowly like a sweet. It gives you nicotine in a similar way to the gum and Microtab.

**Nicotine nasal spray** is the fastest acting form of NRT available. The nicotine gets into the body through the lining of the nose. Nicotine taken in this way is absorbed quickly.

**Inhalator (E-cigarette)** is a plastic device, containing a battery-operated element, shaped like a cigarette with a nicotine cartridge fitted into it. Sucking on the mouthpiece (vaping) releases nicotine vapour, which gets absorbed through your mouth and throat. Potentially their widespread use by existing tobacco smokers could significantly reduce tobacco usage. However, their use by young non-smokers is possibly perpetuating the attractions and lure of smoking in the population and re-normalising smoking.

## Contraindications to NRT

NRT should be used with care in the following groups and only where benefit is considered to outweigh risk:

- patients who weigh <45 kg must always use the lower dose forms of NRT.
- patients with recent or planned angioplasty, bypass grafting or stenting.
- patients with unstable angina.
- pregnant or lactating women, however, there is recent evidence that NRT may be used in pregnancy where there has been failure to quit using other approaches.

**Varenicline** (Champix) available on prescription. Works by reducing craving for a cigarette and by reducing the effects of nicotine. It binds with high affinity and selectivity at the α4β2 neuronal nicotinic acetylcholine receptor, where it acts as a partial agonist. Its binding both alleviates symptoms of craving and withdrawal, and reduces the rewarding and reinforcing effects of smoking by preventing nicotine binding to α4β2 receptors. Varenicline usage may be associated with nausea and other gastrointestinal disorders such as vomiting. It should normally be prescribed only as part of a programme of behavioural support. Smokers should set a date to stop smoking and treatment with Varenicline should start 1 to 2 weeks before this date. Treatment normally lasts for 12 weeks.

**Bupropion** (Zyban) available on prescription, should only be prescribed as an adjunct to a programme of support. Start tablets 1 or 2 weeks before quitting. Side effects include insomnia, dry mouth, neuro-psychiatric disorders, convulsions, hypertension and gastro-intestinal upsets.

**References:**

➢ NICE technology appraisal guidance 123. Varenicline for smoking cessation. National Institute for Health and Clinical Excellence, 2007. www.nice.org.uk/TA123

➢ Why e-cigarettes are dividing the public health community BMJ 2015; 350:h3317

➢ Stead LF Nicotine replacement therapy for smoking cessation. Cochrane Database Syst Rev. 2012 Nov 14; 11:CD000146

**ARRANGE:** Ensure follow-up contact.

It is important to arrange further follow-up and support, either with a GP, referral to a specialist clinic, or by telephone, and this is the final step with patients willing to quit.

Follow up visits significantly increase the rates of smoking cessation. Initial follow-up should begin soon after the quit date, preferably during the first week because the first week is the most vulnerable time for smokers who have quit. A second follow-up contact is recommended within the first month. But additional appointments can be scheduled as appropriate and in discussion with the patient.

During follow-up problems already encountered should be identified and challenges in the immediate future anticipated.

Also assess medication use and problems, and continue to encourage and support the patient.

Always address tobacco use at next clinic visit. Congratulate abstinent patients on their success. If tobacco use has occurred, review circumstances and elicit a recommitment to total abstinence.

### 5.15 Patients not ready to make an attempt to quit

Patients who are unwilling to make a quit attempt at this time may respond to brief motivational interventions (directive, patient centred counselling), which may be effective in increasing future quit attempts.

Motivational interviewing techniques focus on exploring the smoker's feelings, beliefs, ideas, and values regarding smoking in an effort to uncover any ambivalence about using tobacco, and identify potential barriers (such as fear of failure, the pleasure from smoking).

You can get patient to think about quitting by asking questions:

*What do you like about smoking?*
*What don't you like about smoking?*
*What do you gain from smoking?*
*What would you lose by quitting?*
*What are the triggers that make you want to smoke?*

The likes and dislikes of smoking can be explored using a decision balance table. This tool can highlight discrepancy between a patient's behaviour and their values.

You can ask your patient to take the table home to complete the exercise.

You can also ask the patient to complete the Smoking Motives Questionnaire which will also help them to explore their smoking behaviour.

Having the patient use his or her own words to explore his/her smoking behaviour and commit to change is more effective than clinician exhortations, lectures, or arguments for quitting which tend to build, rather than lessen, patient resistance to change.

Give the smoker some written information on the risks of smoking and the benefits of quitting and ask permission to talk about smoking again sometime in the future.

**Reference:**

➤ The Wisconsin Inventory of Smoking Dependence Motives
http://www.ctri.wisc.edu/Researchers/AcceptedWISDMManuscript.pdf

### 5.15.1 Smoking Motives Questionnaire

This set of questions will help you to think about why you smoke and what you might miss most if you quit.

1.  Do you use smoking to help you cope with stress?

Yes very much

Yes quite a bit

Yes a little

Not really

Not at all

2.  Do you use smoking to help you socialise?

Yes very much

Yes quite a bit

Yes a little

Not really

Not at all

3.  Do you use smoking to give you something to do when you are bored?

Yes very much

Yes quite a bit

Yes a little

Not really

Not at all

4.  Do you use smoking to help you concentrate and stay alert?

Yes very much

Yes quite a bit

Yes a little

Not really

Not at all

5. Do you smoke because you feel uncomfortable if you don't?

Yes very much

Yes quite a bit

Yes a little

Not really

Not at all

6. Do you use smoking to help you keep your weight down?

Yes very much

Yes quite a bit

Yes a little

Not really

Not at all

7. Do you enjoy smoking?

Yes very much

Yes quite a bit

Yes a little

Not really

Not at all

**Reference:**

➢ Smoking Motives Questionnaire NHS Centre for Smoking Cessation & Training

http://www.ncsct.co.uk/publication_motivation-to-stop-smoking.php

## 5.15.2 Smoking: Decisional Balance

The following statements represent different opinions about smoking. Please rate HOW IMPORTANT each statement is to your decision to smoke according to the following five point scale:

**1 = Not important**

**2 = Slightly important**

**3 = Moderately important**

**4 = Very important**

**5 = Extremely important**

1. Smoking cigarettes is pleasurable.
2. My smoking affects the health of others.
3. I like the image of a cigarette smoker.
4. Others close to me would suffer if I became ill from smoking.
5. I am relaxed and therefore more pleasant when smoking.
6. Because I continue to smoke some people think I lack the character to quit.
7. If I try to stop smoking I shall become irritable and a pain to be around.
8. Smoking cigarettes is hazardous to my health.
9. My family and friends like me better when I am happy smoking than when I am miserably trying to quit.
10. I'm embarrassed to have to smoke.
11. I like myself better when I smoke.
12. My cigarette smoking bothers other people.
13. Smoking helps me concentrate and do better work.
14. People think I'm foolish for ignoring the warnings about cigarette smoking.

15. Smoking cigarettes relieves tension.
16. People close to me disapprove of my smoking.
17. By continuing to smoke I feel I am making my own decisions.
18. I'm foolish to ignore the warnings about smoking.
19. After not smoking for a while a cigarette makes me feel great.
20. I would be more energetic right now if I did not smoke.

**Scoring**

Total separately the values for pros and cons and see which preponderates.

PROS      1,3,5,7,9,11,13,15,17,19 (odd numbers)

CONS     2,4,6,8,10,12,14,16,18,20 (even numbers)

**Reference:**

➢ Velicer, W.F., Diclemente C.C., Prochaska J.O., & Brandenburg N. (1985). Decisional balance measure for assessing and predicting smoking status. Journal of Personality and Social Psychology, 48, 1279-1289

### 5.16 Barriers to discussing smoking with patients

Lastly, you may have some concerns about discussing smoking with patients, such as:

- Lack of time.
- Interventions as brief as 3 minutes can increase cessation rates significantly.
- Concern that smoking cessation knowledge and skills are insufficient and lack of good resources to back-up counselling.

- There are relevant clinical guidelines which you can consult or special training courses for health workers which you could attend.
- Doubts about the effectiveness of advice.
- Fear of damaging the relationship with the patient.

Generally, patients feel that GP advice regarding smoking is acceptable and appropriate and smokers cite a physician's advice to quit as an important motivator to stop smoking.

- Intermittent contact with individual patients.
- Patients do not want to hear about quitting smoking.

**Remember:**

**Smokers may expect to be asked about their smoking. If the issue is not addressed many could assume that smoking is OK.**

**Reference:**

➤ Stead Factors influencing European GPs' engagement in smoking cessation: a multi-country literature review Br J Gen Pract 2009 Sep 59 (566):682-690

Here is another opportunity to role play with your colleagues. Role play for about 15-20 minutes.

### Smoking: Brief Intervention - let us try it!

Joe is a 52 year old construction worker. He has smoked 20 cigarettes a day for about 30 years. He scores 6 on the Fagerström Test for Nicotine Dependence. He usually has a cigarette with tea as soon as he awakes. He has presented to you on 3 occasions in the last 6 months with symptoms of acute bronchitis - productive cough, breathless, wheezy. He mentions he is getting breathless and wheezy sometimes when climbing ladders or carrying heavy loads.

With a colleague, one of you pretend to be Joe and the other the primary care doctor. Go through the 5As with Joe.

### In Summary

In this chapter we have considered the modifiable CVD risk factor smoking. We have outlined why it is relevant to the topic of cardiovascular health, and given some data about the nature and size of the problem in the UK and Scotland. Our aim has been to promote the cardiovascular health of your patients by educating them about the risks of smoking. We have revised the increased risks of developing CVD from smoking.

- We have shown how you can assess a patient's dependence on tobacco and willingness to quit smoking.
- We have given you some tools to assess the patient's level of smoking.
- We have also focused on the matter of behaviour change, and how to assess a patient's readiness to change.
- We have described the 5 As - a brief intervention which you can try in order to support a patient to stop smoking.
- We have given you details of smoking cessation adjuncts, including pharmacological interventions which have been shown to be successful in helping someone stop smoking.

# 6. Alcohol

## Key Points

- Excessive consumption of alcohol is a significant risk factor for development of CVD, hepatic cirrhosis and liver cancer.
- Your aim is to be able to improve the cardiovascular health of your patients by educating them about the risks relating to alcohol.

**Objectives**:

- To revise the increased risks of CVD from alcohol.
- To be able to take an accurate alcohol consumption history from a patient.
- To know more detail about brief behavioural interventions for alcohol.
- To commence behavioural change and lifestyle modification in your patients.

We now will consider the topic of alcohol in relation to CVD prevention. We are going to examine why this topic is relevant to CVD. We are also going to look at specific data we have on this particular health behaviour in the UK.

Then we will focus in greater detail on how to establish your patient's alcohol consumption behaviour and habits. We shall look at some of the international and national guidelines and 'best practice' recommendations for alcohol consumption management.

Lastly, we will offer you some practical advice on how to administer brief interventions in the community setting to encourage your patient to change to a more healthy lifestyle and behaviour, using evidence based techniques.

## 6.1 Alcohol - The Facts Revised

In chapter 3 we looked at the non-modifiable and modifiable risk factors for CVD prevention. One of the modifiable risk factors is alcohol. Let us revise the facts.

- A male drinking more than 8 units a day will double his risk of developing coronary heart disease.
- A female drinking more than 6 units a day will increase her risk of developing coronary heart disease by a factor of 1.3.
- Episodic drinking of more than 8 units over a short period of time significantly increases the risk of developing CVD.
- Alcohol is a significant cause of hypertension, arrhythmias, and cardiomyopathies, leading to coronary heart disease, as well as strokes. The risk of developing cancers, including hepatic & breast cancer, is increased by drinking alcohol.
- Heavy or binge drinking (more than 8 units for men and 6 units for women per day) increases the risk of sudden cardiac deaths and arrhythmias by 45%.

- Women over the age of 55 years may get a small reduction in CVD risk if they drink up to 5 units of alcohol weekly.

A common problem in Eastern European countries is drinking cheap surrogate alcohol products such as perfume, detergents or industrial cleaning products. This is especially harmful, with some reports suggesting a much higher association with mortality than with pure beverage alcohol. The more often surrogate alcohol is drunk, the stronger the association with mortality, irrespective of the volume or amount consumed. The products contain very high concentrations of ethanol and there have been suggestions that the high concentration of ethanol in the blood over repeated episodes is what causes the greater damage to the body.

**References:**

➤ M Gronbaek et al. Type of alcohol consumed and mortality from all causes, coronary heart disease, and cancer. Annals of Internal Medicine 2000 133: 411-419

➤ M Marmot. Alcohol & Coronary Artery Disease, Int. J. Epidemiol. (2001) 30 (4): 724-729.

➤ D Leon et al Hazardous alcohol drinking and premature mortality in Russia: a population based case-control study The Lancet, Volume 369, Issue 9578, Pages 2001 - 2009, 16 June 2007

➤ British Heart Foundation Beating Heart Disease Together 2012

➤ Filmore et al Moderate alcohol use and reduced mortality risk Annals Epidemiology 17 (5, Supplement 1) S16-S23

➤ Department of Health UK Chief Medical Officer's Alcohol Guidelines Review Jan 2016

## 6.2 Alcohol in England

- In 2009 men in England consumed 15.6 units of alcohol weekly.
- Over nine million people in England drink more than recommended levels of alcohol.
- 2 million men and 1 million women drink hazardous levels of alcohol.
- In 2010/11 there were 200,000 hospital admissions for alcohol-related illness.
- 1.5% of premature deaths in the UK are alcohol-related. In 2012 there were 6,500 alcohol-related deaths in the UK, a 19% increase since 2001.
- The cost of alcohol-related illness in the UK in 2006/7 was £25 billion, by 2013 this had risen to £35 billion.
- Older people drink alcohol more frequently than younger, but when younger people drink they drink more heavily.
- Alcohol liver disease in young and middle aged increased by six times in the past 30 years, although there has been a decrease in alcohol consumption since 2005.

**References:**

➢ British Heart Foundation CHD Statistics in England 2012
➢ Statistics on Alcohol England NHS Information Centre 2012
➢ British Society of Gastroenterology, British Association for study of Liver & Alcohol Health Alliance - Alcohol related disease 2010
➢ Alcohol Concern Statistics on alcohol 2015

### 6.2.1 Alcohol and CVD in Scotland

- Alcohol contributes to 1 in 20 deaths in Scotland - double the rate in England.
- In 2010 in Scotland 26% of men and 16% of women were reported to regularly binge drink.
- Premature mortality rates are 25% higher in Scotland than in England.
- Mortality rates are 89% higher in socially deprived areas.
- In 2010 CVD was the main cause of death in Scotland.
- In 2010 there were >8000 deaths from CHD and 12,000 heart attacks (7000 in men and 5000 in women).
- More than 270,000 people in Scotland had CHD and over 200,000 had angina.
- In 2014 alcohol sales had fallen by 9% from 2009 levels.
- In 2014 23% men and 17% women drank alcohol at harmful or hazardous levels.
- The cost of alcohol-related disease in Scotland was £3.6 billion in 2014.

**References:**

- British Heart Foundation CHD Statistics in Scotland 2012
- Chest Heart & Stroke Scotland Response to Alcohol (Minimum Pricing) (Scotland) Bill 2012
- Alcohol Focus Scotland Alcohol facts and figures 2015

### 6.3 Licensing Laws in the UK

**Existing:**

These regulate the sale and consumption of alcohol.

Pubs, restaurants and shops must be licensed to sell alcohol.

To drink on the premises requires an on-licence.

To sell alcohol to take away requires an off-licence.

Alcohol can only be purchased by people over the age of 18 years.

**Proposed:**

Imposing a minimum unit price (mup) for alcohol, possibly 45-50 pence per unit.

It is estimated a minimum price of 45p per unit would result in an annual savings to the NHS of £220 million.

It has been shown that, irrespective of income, moderate drinkers would be little affected by mup. Harmful drinkers would gain the greatest beneficial effects.

**References:**

➤ Licensing Act 2003

➤ Holmes Effects of minimum unit pricing for alcohol on different income & socioeconomic groups Lancet doi:10.1016/S0140-6736(13)62417-4

## 6.4 Why do People Drink Alcohol?

Socially accepted part of our culture.

Advertising and promotion.

Peer example and influences.

Accompanying food.

Coping with stress.

Assisting relaxing.

Improving mood.

Increasing courage.

Low self-esteem.

Promoting a different image.

Proving something to one's self and others.

**Reference:**

➢ http://alcohol.addictionblog.org/why-do-people-start-drinking-alcohol-top-10-reasons 2015

## 6.5 Assessing Alcohol Consumption

In taking an alcohol history, what questions should you ask your patients about their drinking of alcohol?

Consider why might it be difficult for the patient to talk about or admit to the amount of alcohol they drink (for example culture-dependent or because alcohol usage is known to be bad).

Here is a comprehensive list of questions a clinician can ask a patient in order to determine whether their alcohol consumption and habits exceed recommended amounts and practice:

*Do you drink alcohol?*

*How often do you drink alcohol?*

*In general, what sort of alcohol do you drink (e.g. beer, wine, vodka)?*

*On average, how much alcohol do you drink in one sitting?*

*Do you have alcohol-free days?*

*Have there been times that you have drunk more alcohol, on average, than you are drinking now?*

*What do you think about your alcohol consumption (e.g. is it too much)?*

*Have you, or anyone in your life, ever been concerned about the amount of alcohol that you drink?*

*Do you drink any alcohol substitutes?*

## 6.6 Measuring Alcohol Consumption

Units of alcohol are used to quantify the amount of alcohol consumed. Benefits include standardisation for use internationally and nationally and ability to measure different types of alcohol consumed.

1 unit = 8g alcohol.

1 unit = volume (litres) x Alcohol by value (ABV= % strength of alcohol).

For example: 75 ml of 40% whisky/vodka (0.075 x 40) = 3 units alcohol.

Recommended upper limits of alcohol in UK:

Female: 2-3 units per day and up to 14 units per week.

Male: 3-4 units per day and up to 21 units per week.

In January 2016 UK Government advised that men **and** women should limit their weekly alcohol consumption to 14 units (one-and-a-half bottles of wine/5 pints of 5% abv lager). No alcohol should be drunk during pregnancy.

Do you think that your patients would, on the whole, be able to conform to these limits?

## How many units in a drink?

1 unit = (125 ml) glass of lower strength (12%) wine or champagne, small bottle (275 ml) of lower strength (4%) alcopop, half pint of lower strength (4%) lager, beer or cider, single measure of spirit (40%).

2 units = standard glass (175 ml) of lower strength (12%) wine or champagne, pint of lower strength (4%) lager, beer or cider, 440 ml can of medium strength (4.5%) lager, beer or cider, double measure of spirit (40%).

3 units = pint medium strength (5%) lager, beer or cider, large glass (250 ml) of lower strength (12%) wine, large bottle (700 ml) of lower strength (4%) alcopop.

4 units = large bottle (700 ml) higher strength (5.5%) alcopop, 500 ml can of higher strength (7.5%) lager, beer or cider.

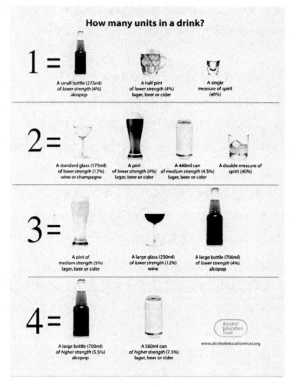

**Reference:**

➤ http://www.drinkingandyou.com/site/pix/middle/illust/how%20many.gif

### 6.7 Tools for Assessment of Alcohol Consumption
### Alcohol Use Disorders Identification Test (AUDIT)

A very useful validated tool for assessing the risk associated with your patient's alcohol consumption comprising 10 questions. Sensitivity of 92% and Specificity of 94%.

AUDIT-C is a shortened version comprising the first 3 questions of AUDIT. The shortened form has only a Sensitivity of 86% and Specificity of 72%.

## 6.7.1 AUDIT - C Test

How often do you have a drink containing alcohol?

a. never

b. monthly or less

c. 2-4 times a month

d. 2-3 times a week

e. 4 or more times a week

How many standard drinks do you have a day?

a. 1-2

b. 3-4

c. 5-6

d. 7-9

e. 10 or more

How often do you have 6 or more drinks on one occasion?

a. never

b. less than monthly

c. monthly

d. weekly

e. daily or most days

The scoring system is: a=0, b=1, c=2, d=3, e=4.

The test is positive for excessive alcohol if men score >4 and women >3.

If a patient scores more than 4 or 3, then they are probably engaging in excessive or hazardous drinking, and this should trigger a discussion with the clinician about their alcohol consumption and lifestyle.

A score of >8 suggests hazardous or harmful alcohol use.

**Reference:**

➢ Saunders, J.B., and Aasland, O.G. WHO Collaborative Project on the Identification and Treatment of Persons with Harmful Alcohol Consumption. Report on Phase I: Development of a Screening Instrument. Geneva: World Health Organization, 1987

### 6.7.2 Assessing Readiness for Change
### The Stages of Change

Let us apply the Prochaska/Di Clementi Transtheoretical model of change (See CVD Risk Factors and Primary Prevention chapter 3).

Pre-contemplation/Contemplation/Preparation/Action/Maintenance.

**Reference:**

➢ Prochaska Stages of change & decisional balance for 12 problem behaviours Health Psychol 1994; 13:39-46

➢ Prochaska & Di Clemente The Transtheoretical approach Handbook of psychotherapy integration OUP 2005 147-171

### 6.7.3 Brief Interventions for Alcohol Consumption

Once you have established that a patient is drinking alcohol excessively, you can implement in the primary care setting a brief intervention lasting 5-20 minutes. There is good evidence this will result in a reduction of alcohol consumption and fewer episodes of binge drinking, with the effect lasting for up to one year and maybe longer.

This can be undertaken when the opportunity arises. It is most effective if the patient is helped to consider their perceived benefit from a reduction in consumption and the disadvantages of maintaining their current drinking pattern. The ideal outcome of the brief Intervention is setting some agreed goals for reduction of consumption, or abstinence.

### Brief Intervention - a Tool

Let us consider the constituent elements of the process.

**Feedback** – about personal risk of current consumption levels. The clinician can inform their patient about how their drinking may be harmful, and how their personal habit compares to national or international recommendations. This is more effective if you tailor your information-giving to the patient's individual habits.

**Responsibility** – emphasise personal responsibility to change – a patient needs to be engaged with the process of change in order to sustain a change in behaviour.

**Advice** – to cut down or abstain based on risk/consumption – again tailor according to consumption and habit.

**Menu** – of alternative options – the longest part of the consultation, where there is discussion about what and how behaviours can change.

**Empathy** – from clinician with attentive listening and gentle encouragement, rather than directive or confrontational style.

**Self-efficacy** – help the patient believe that they have the ability to change, that it is within their power to change, by making small steps and working towards achievable and realistic goals.

**References:**

> Scottish Intercollegiate Guidelines Network
  http://www.sign.ac.uk/guidelines/fulltext/74/section3.html.

> A cross-national trial of brief interventions with heavy drinkers. WHO Brief Intervention Study Group. Am J Public Health 1996; 86(7):948-55.

> Moyer A, Finney JW, Swearingen CE, Vergun P. Brief interventions for alcohol problems: a meta-analytic review of controlled investigations in treatment-seeking and non-treatment-seeking populations. Addiction 2002; 97(3):279-92

> Fleming MF, Barry KL, Manwell LB, Johnson K, London R. Brief physician advice for problem alcohol drinkers. A randomized controlled trial in community-based primary care practices. JAMA 1997; 277(13):1039-45

## 6.8 Setting Goals for Change

This will be most successful if done in collaboration with the patient. Stepwise reduction is often most effective. Give practical advice, such as, *Alternating soft drinks with alcohol, Not entering into rounds* (where each person in the group takes turns to buy a drink for everyone else in the group) and *Refraining from going to venues where drinking normally occurs.*

Monitor and review regularly and offer details of local support services, agencies and charities. Joining organisations such as Alcohol Anonymous may be helpful.

**Reference:**
- ➤ Stretcher V et al Goal setting as a strategy for health behavior change Health Educ Q. 1995 May; 22(2):190-200

## 6.9 Pharmacological Aids

**Nalmefene** an opioid receptor modulator reduces alcohol craving and thus consumption. Dosage one 18mgm tablet when required. Numerous gastro-intestinal and cardiovascular side effects have been reported, although all are uncommon. It is too early to assess the part it will play in management of alcoholics and, if used, should be as an adjunct to counselling. It is available on NHS prescription in Scotland.

**References:**
- ➤ Alcohol-Use Disorders: Diagnosis, Assessment and Management of Harmful Drinking and Alcohol Dependence Pharmacological aids NICE Clinical Guidelines, No. 115

> K Mann et al Extending Treatment Options in Alcohol Dependence: A randomized controlled study of as-needed Nalmefene Biol Psych Vol 73, Issue 8 (April 15 2013)

## 6.10 Monitoring Alcohol Consumption

Transdermal alcohol concentrations in sweat accurately reflect blood alcohol concentrations. A study is being undertaken in the UK to determine whether transdermal alcohol bracelets can be used to monitor alcohol intake in drivers convicted of alcohol related driving offences.

**Reference:**

> Hawthorne Transdermal alcohol measurement 2006 Canadian Soc Forensic Science Jour 39(2):65-71

## Alcohol: Brief Intervention - let's try it

Here is a clinical scenario:

Alex (a man or a woman) is 45 years old. He/she works on the railways, 5 sometimes 6 days a week. He/she is divorced and has 2 children aged 8 and 11, who he/she sees at the weekend every other week. Alex drinks on average 5 times a week. Twice a week work colleagues go out for a drink. Twice a week he/she drinks with a friend in a local bar. Once a week he/she drinks with the family when they have a meal together. He/she drinks beer or wine. Usually about 2 pints of beer, but, with his/her friend and family drinks 1/2 bottle of wine during a meal. His/her father died at the age of 63 from a heart attack and his/her sister has diabetes.

This is an opportunity to role play with a colleague. One of you pretends to be Alex. The other of your pair needs to act as a Primary care physician. Have a conversation, for 5 minutes, about Alex's drinking habits. Try a brief intervention!

**Summary - have you met your aim and objectives?**

Now consider your aims and objectives at the start of this chapter and whether they have been achieved.

**Aim**

To be able to promote the cardiovascular health of your patients by educating them about alcohol.

**Objectives:**
- To revise the risks of developing CVD from consuming alcohol.
- To be able to take an accurate alcohol consumption history from a patient.
- To know in more detail about brief behavioural interventions for alcohol.
- To commence behavioural change and lifestyle modification in your patients.

We have compared the problems of alcohol in the UK and Scotland and highlighted some common problems, some similarities and some differences.

# 7. Diet and Weight

## Key Points

- There is a direct relationship between increased weight and CVD risk.
- Being overweight increases one's chances of developing many illnesses.
- When dieting first change how much you eat, then change what you eat.

Your aim is to be able to improve the cardiovascular health of your patients by educating them about the risks relating to unhealthy diet and obesity.

We now will consider the topics of diet and obesity in relation to CVD prevention.

**Objectives:**

- To revise the increased risks of CVD from unhealthy diet and obesity.
- To be able to take an accurate dietary history from a patient.
- To know more detail about how healthy eating and weight reduction can improve cardiovascular health and how to talk to patients about the topic.

## 7.1 Diet and Obesity

## 7.1.1 The Healthy Nutrition Pyramid

Oils

Fats Sweets

Meat Poultry Fish

Eggs Milk Cheese Yogurt

Fruits                    Vegetables

Bread Cereals            Rice Pasta

This diagram was originally developed as part of the WHO Healthy Nutrition initiative. You can see that it provides, in graphic form, an outline of relative proportions of foods and food groups which should be eaten to maintain a healthy diet.

At the top the smallest part of our diet should be fats, oils and sweet foods. The greatest part of our diet should consist of non-refined carbohydrates such as brown bread, cereals and grains, legumes and beans. Fruit and vegetables ought to provide a large component of one's diet, and animal foods such as meat and eggs should only provide a small proportion of what is eaten on a daily basis.

WHO has stated that consuming more than 45g of protein a day, and fewer than 400gm of fruit and vegetables a day, are considered to be unhealthy practices. The proportion of fat intake compared to other food groups should not exceed 30% of the total caloric intake, and more than 20g of alcohol a day is unhealthy. The recommended total daily energy consumption for a man is 2500 calories, and for a woman 2000 calories.

**Reference:**
> Food Pyramids & Health. What should you really eat? Harvard School of Public Health 2012


### 7.1.2 WHO/CINDI Principles of Healthy Nutrition

In 1999 the WHO developed some principles of healthy eating and nutrition, and these were adopted by the CINDI (Countrywide Integrated Non-communicable Disease Intervention) programme. These recommendations provide a basic model which can be adapted according to local and cultural traditions, eating habits and foods.

The 12 principles include:
- Eat a variety of foods originating mainly from plants, not animals.
- Eat 400mgm of vegetables and fruit (preferably fresh) a day.
- Ensure that fat does not contribute to more than 30% of daily caloric intake.
- Replace saturated fat, such as fatty/red meat with unsaturated fats, such as beans, legumes, fish, lean meat and poultry.
- Use low-fat and low-salt milk products.

- Total salt intake should not exceed one teaspoon (6mgm) daily including salt added in foods such as bread, cured and preserved foods.
- Prepare food in a healthy way, for example steam, bake or boil foods, do not roast or fry.
- Limit alcohol to a maximum of 2 drinks a day (each containing <10 gm alcohol).

So, these are the principles of healthy eating that we and our patients all need to be working towards. But how can we encourage patients to change their nutritional behaviour?

The Academy of Medical Royal Colleges have called for a series of cost-effective regulatory interventions to reduce obesity. Banning marketing of unhealthy foods on television before 9 pm, introducing a 20% tax on sugar sweetened drinks, developing more green spaces for exercise, improving nutritional standards in schools, reducing proximity of fast food outlets to schools and changing nutritional standards in hospitals and the wider food market.

The Mediterranean diet, consisting largely of fruit and vegetables, nuts, fish and olive oil is considered to be cardio-protective.

**Reference:**

> Rashid Time to get Mediterranean with our dietary advice Br Jr Gen Pract 2014 doi: 10.3399/bjgp14X677365

## 7.2 Diet and Obesity - The Facts Revised

Several American and European studies have shown that eating 5 portions of fruit and vegetables a day can reduce the risks of coronary heart disease and stroke. Those who ate 5 portions daily had a risk reduction of 20% compared to those who ate fewer than 3 portions daily. These studies include a longitudinal study which followed 110,000 men and women for 14 years in Harvard, USA. Recent studies have proposed that eating 7-10 portions a day is even more effective, however, it is probably not realistic to expect many individuals to follow that advice.

Whilst all fruit and vegetables are healthy, some in particular have been shown to be especially beneficial. For example dark green vegetables such as spinach, lettuce, greens, cruciferous vegetables such as broccoli, cauliflower, cabbage and citrus fruits such as oranges, lemons, grapefruits.

Two well-reputed studies have also shown that eating a diet rich in fruit and vegetables and low in all fats, but especially saturated and trans fats, can help reduce blood pressure, which in itself is a risk factor for CVD. (Saturated fats come from animals and are present in red meat and dairy foods including cheese, butter and milk. Trans fats are hydrogenated vegetable fats found in baked goods such as cakes, pies, biscuits).

A diet high in saturated or trans fats can lead to high cholesterol levels, which is a high risk factor for CVD.

We also know that being overweight increases one's chances of developing many illnesses including hypertension, high cholesterol, diabetes and other conditions such as some cancers and osteoarthritis. Being obese (in other words having a body mass index greater than 30) significantly increases risk of CVD.

The distribution of fat in the body is a factor. Those who carry their fat more centrally around their abdomen and waists have a greater risk of CVD.

A diet high in sugars and salt can also lead to an increased risk of developing CVD.

**References:**

- ➢ Hung HC, Joshipura KJ, Jiang R, et al. Fruit and vegetable intake and risk of major chronic disease. Natl Cancer Inst. 2004; 96:1577–84
- ➢ He FJ, Nowson CA, Lucas M, MacGregor GA. Increased consumption of fruit and vegetables is related to a reduced risk of coronary heart disease: meta-analysis of cohort studies. J Hum Hypertens. 2007; 21:717–28
- ➢ He FJ, Nowson CA, MacGregor GA. Fruit and vegetable consumption and stroke: meta-analysis of cohort studies. Lancet. 2006; 367:320–26
- ➢ Appel LJ, Moore TJ, Obarzanek E, et al. A clinical trial of the effects of dietary patterns on blood pressure. DASH Collaborative Research Group. N Engl J Med. 1997; 336:1117–24

➢ Appel LJ, Sacks FM, Carey VJ, et al. Effects of protein, monounsaturated fat, and carbohydrate intake on blood pressure and serum lipids: results of the OmniHeart randomized trial. JAMA. 2005; 294:2455–64

## 7.3 Diet and Obesity in the UK

- Since 1994 male obesity (>30 BMI) in the UK has increased from 14% to 22%, female from 17% to 24% and in children from 11% to 16%.
- 38% of adults in the UK had a raised waist circumference in 2009 compared with 23% in 1993.
- Between 1993 and 2012 the proportion of obese men had increased from 13.2% to 24.4% and obese women from 16.4% to 25.1%.
- The proportion of men with raised waist circumference had increased from 20% to 34% and of women from 26% to 45%.
- In 2012/13 the proportion of obese children in Reception class (aged 4-5 years) had fallen marginally to 9.3% from 9.5% in 2011/12 and 9.9% in 2006/07.
- However, in 2012/13 in year 6 (aged 10-11 years) 18.9% of children were obese compared with 19.2% in 2011/12 and 17.5% in 2006/07.
- In 2009/10 poor diet-related illness cost the UK £5.8 billion.
- There is a direct relationship between increased weight and CVD risk.

**References:**

➢ National Obesity Observatory NHS Jan 2011

➢ Economic burden of ill-health due to diet, physical activity, smoking, alcohol, obesity in the UK 2006-7 Scarborough et al J Pub Health 1093/pubmed/fdr033

➢ British Heart Foundation CHD statistics in England 2012

➢ Statistics on obesity, physical activity & diet in England 2011 and 2014 NHS Health & Social Care Information Centre

### 7.3.1 Diet and Obesity in Scotland

- Between 1995 and 2010 the proportion of overweight adults in Scotland increased from 52% to 64%. By 2014 this had increased to 65%.

- In 2010 >25% men and women were obese. In 2014 28% were obese. This has increased since 1995 from 16% of men and 17% of women.

- Childhood obesity appears to be levelling off. In 2010, 32% of children in Scotland had a BMI above the healthy range. In 2014, 31% of children were obese, 4% of boys and 28% of girls.

- In 2010 in Scotland 20% men and 23% women consumed 5 portions of fruit and vegetables a day.

- 15% of their energy came from saturated fats (recommended maximum <10%).

- Consumption of fruit and vegetables was lower in Scotland than in England and Wales.

- In Scotland a higher proportion of men and women are overweight/obese than in England.
- There are many similarities between the unhealthy diet and high alcohol consumption and high CVD risk in Russia and Scotland (particularly in western regions and parts of Glasgow).

**References:**
➤ Scottish Health Survey 2013 and 2014
➤ Health of Scotland's Population - Healthy Weight 2011
➤ Scarborough et al Differences in CHD, stroke & cancer mortality rates in England, Wales, Scotland & N Ireland BMJ Open 2011; 1e000263

## 7.4 Obesity and Psychiatric Disorders

There is an increased incidence of depression, dysthymia, mania and hypomania in obese and extremely obese individuals, more marked in women than men.

Individuals suffering from depression, anxiety and eating disorders, such as anorexia nervosa, may have difficulty in controlling food consumption, taking adequate exercise and maintaining healthy weight.

**References:**
➤ Barry Obesity & Psychiatric Disorders Psychiatric Times Dec 2009
➤ Collins Behavioural & Psychological Factors in Obesity Jour Lancester Gen Hosp Winter 2009 Vol 4, No 4

## 7.5 Why do People Overeat?

Parental influence and desire to please mother.

Psychological problems, such as depression, anxiety or stress.

Comfort.

Peer influence and social pressures.

Enjoyment of foods.

Food addiction.

Cultural factors.

Boredom.

Habit and mindlessness.

Genetic.

This is not a comprehensive list and you may wish to add your own reasons.

**Reference:**

> ➢ Jade D Compulsive Eating & Binge Eating Disorder National Centre for Eating disorders 2010

## 7.6 Diet: Assessing Diet and Weight

Take a focused history.

*How many times a week do you eat red meat?*
*How much of foods containing saturated fat do you eat per week?*
*How many portions of fruit and vegetable do you eat a day?*
*Do you cook with salt and eat cured, preserved or processed foods?*
*How much refined sugar do you eat each week?*

Of course the simplest way to assess weight is to weigh someone! But this doesn't take into account how tall they are, so a person with a height of 1.8m might weight the same as a person who is 1.4m but for the former person this is a healthy weight and for the latter it is not.

**BMI** (Mass in Kg/Height in $m^{2)}$ is a better measure of weight because it takes into account a person's height as well. BMI of 20-25 is healthy. However there are some occasions when it might not reveal the whole picture. For example, muscle is heavier than fat, so a person with big muscle bulk may be found to have a high BMI, even though their body fat content is low.

A low BMI of less than 20 confers its own health risks, for example, it can interfere with a woman's menstrual cycle and be a factor in subsequent fertility or lead to a reduction in bone density.

**References:**
> NBHLI. The Practical Guide for Identification, Evaluation, and Treatment of Overweight and Obesity in Adults. 2000.
> Working Group on Monitoring Scottish Dietary Targets Workshop, September 2003

## 7.7 Distribution of Body Fat

Studies have shown that how a person's fat is distributed is associated with cardiovascular risk. People whose fat is distributed centrally in the abdomen have a higher risk. Waist measurement has therefore become a useful way of assessing risk. Increased waist circumference can be a marker for increased risk, even in persons of normal weight.

To correctly measure your waist, stand and place a tape measure around your middle, just above your hipbones. Measure your waist just after you breathe out.

### 7.7.1 Obesity - Waist Measurements

|  | Increased risk | High risk |
|---|---|---|
| Men not Asian | 94-101 cm | >= 102 cm |
| Men-Asian | - | >= 90 cm |
| Women-not Asian | 80-87 cm | >= 88 cm |
| Women-Asian | - | >= 80 cm |

This table shows the level of risk associated with waist measurement. You will notice that among people of Asian ethnic background high risk is associated with lower waist measurements.

### 7.7.2 Classification of Overweight and Obesity by BMI
### Waist circumference and associated disease risks
### Disease Risk* relative to normal weight & waist circumference

|  | BMI (kg/m$^2$) | Obesity Class | Men 102cm (40in) or less Women 88cm (35in) or less | Men > 102cm Women >88cm |
|---|---|---|---|---|
| Underweight | <18.5 |  |  |  |
| Normal | 18.5-24.9 |  |  |  |
| Overweight | 25-29.9 |  | Increased | High |
| Obesity | 30-34.9 | I | High | Very High |
|  | 5-39.9 | II | Very High | Very High |
| Extreme Obesity | 40+ | III | Extremely High | Extremely High |

* Disease risk for type 2 diabetes, hypertension, CVD

**Reference:**

> http://www.health.gov/dietaryguidelines/dga2005/healthieryou/html/chapt er4.html 2005

## 7.8 Metabolic Syndrome

Metabolic syndrome affects one in four adults in the UK.

## Diagnosis

Waist circumference of 37 inches (92.5cm) or more (European men) or 31.5 inches (78.75cm) or more (European and South Asian women).

Waist circumference of 35.5 (88.75cm) inches or more (South Asian men).

High levels of triglycerides and low levels of HDL.

Blood pressure consistently above 140/90mmHg.

Insulin resistance (inability to control blood sugar levels).

Increased risk of developing deep vein thrombosis (DVT).

Tendency to develop inflammatory conditions.

## Causes

Genetic tendency towards insulin resistance.

Overweight.

Physically inactive.

Metabolic syndrome is especially common in Asian and African-Caribbean people, and in women with polycystic ovary syndrome (PCOS).

**Reference:**

> www.nhlbi.nih.gov/health/health-topics/topics/ms

### 7.9 Changing Diet and Weight

The National Institute of Clinical Excellence in the UK (NICE) develops guidelines for best practice for many clinical domains. Its guidelines for weight management of adults states that a primary care clinician should advise the following approach:

- Help people to assess their weight and aim for a realistic target, meaning an initial weight reduction of 5-10%.
- Aim for a maximum weekly weight loss of 0.5-1 kg.
- Focus on long-term lifestyle changes rather than short-term quick fixes.
- Use a balanced, healthy eating approach.
- Balance changes in diet with increase in amounts of activity or exercise.
- Recommend regular physical activity with practical realistic advice.
- Offer regular and frequent support and monitoring.
- In particular, change what one eats long-term rather than 'going on a diet'.
- Consider with the person potential lapses or 'high risk' situations, and how to cope with them.

**Reference:**

➢ Managing overweight and obesity in adults – lifestyle weight management services NICE guidelines PH53 2014

### 7.9.1 Legislative Changes

The possibility of introducing a tax on foodstuffs and soft drinks containing sugar is under consideration. A recent study in Mexico demonstrated that taxes on sugar-sweetened beverages significantly reduced purchases of taxed beverages. From 2018 a levy on sugar-sweetened drinks will be introduced in the UK. The revenue will be spent on funding sport in primary schools.

**Reference:**
- ➢ Colchero M, et al Beverage purchases from stores in Mexico under the excise tax on sugar sweetened beverages BMJ 2016; 352:h6704

### 7.9.2 Bariatric Surgery

Substantial weight loss and thus prevention of 5000 heart attacks could be achieved if the 1.4 million obese people in the UK undertook bariatric surgery (gastric bypass, sleeve gastrectomy, gastric band).

**Reference:**
- ➢ Ian J. Douglas et al Bariatric Surgery in the United Kingdom: A Cohort Study of Weight Loss and Clinical Outcomes in Routine Clinical Care. PLOS Medicine doi:10.1371/journal.pmed.1001925

### 7.9.3 Changing Eating Behaviour to Lose Weight

The first step is to change how much you eat.

The second step is to change what you eat.

Let us apply the Prochaska/Di Clementi Transtheoretical model of change (See CVD Risk Factors and Primary Prevention - chapter 3) Pre-contemplation/Contemplation/Preparation/Action/Maintenance.

**Reference:**

➢ Hasler G Application of Prochaska's transtheoretical model of change to patients with eating disorders J Psychosom Res. 2004 Jul; 57(1):67-72

### 7.9.4 Changing Diet and Weight - Process

The National Obesity Observatory, which is under the umbrella of the National Health Service in the UK, produced a publication called 'Brief Interventions for Weight Management' in April 2011.

Setting specific and achievable goals at the outset should help achieve behaviour change. It is preferable to focus on short-term goals as they are more realistic and tangible, and less difficult to postpone. Greater likelihood of accomplishment provides quicker rewards and positive reinforcement.

Focus on behaviour change rather than physiological change, for example reducing fat intake rather than reducing cholesterol levels. Behaviour changes are easier to achieve and do not rely on physiological factors which may have a genetic component to them (as, for example, cholesterol does).

Self-monitoring improves effectiveness by allowing the individual to identify progress. This can be done simply by keeping a diary of changes, for example dietary intake or exercise taken, or charting weight loss. This provides an immediate positive feedback.

Promote self-efficacy (meaning an individual's confidence in their ability to achieve specific behaviours).

To do this explore potential barriers – for example asking, *What is stopping you from switching from a piece of chocolate to a piece of fruit a day?,* and considering factors which led to previous successes/failures.

Resist from simply telling the individual what they should do, or how they should change. Instead try to get them to identify changes they can make in their life. Regular monitoring and follow-up provides opportunities for monitoring of weight and other CVD parameters for example blood pressure, feedback, positive reinforcement and encouragement.

**Reference:**
> ➤ Brief Interventions for Weight Management National Obesity Observatory 2011

### 7.9.5 Medication for Chronic Weight Management

In the EU medication such as Orlistat, Naltrexone/Buropion and Liraglutide can be used as adjuncts to assist weight loss. In the USA Phentermine/Topiramate are also available.

**Orlistat** A lipase inhibitor, reduces intestinal fat absorption. One 120mgm capsule taken 1 hour after fatty meals. Side effects steatorrhea and headache. A vitamin supplement should also be taken as absorption of fat solvent vitamins is reduced. Weight loss is modest 2-3 kg a year.

### Diet: Brief Intervention - let's try it!

Another opportunity to role play: Kate/Bill is 56, with a height of 160cm and weight of 80kg. Her/his BMI is 31.6 (= obese). She/he eats 3 meals a day and has snacks of mainly cake or cheese in between meals. She/he eats red meat every day for dinner and lots of potatoes and bread. She/he does not like fruit and tends to have only one piece a day. She/he always has some vegetables with lunch and dinner.

This time in your pair, the one of you who pretended to be the doctor last time should be the patient, and the other person who was the patient last time should be the doctor. Have a conversation for about 5 minutes about Kate/Bill's dietary habits - try a brief intervention!

### Summary - have you met your aim and objectives?

Now consider your aims and objectives at the start of this chapter and whether they have been achieved. You aimed to be able to promote the cardiovascular health of your patients by educating them about diet and obesity.

### Objectives:

- To revise the risks of developing CVD from eating a poor diet.
- To be able to take an accurate dietary history from a patient.
- To know more detail about how healthy eating and weight reduction can improve cardiovascular health and how to talk to patients about the topic.

- To know how to advise your patients to modify their eating habits.

We have compared the problems of unhealthy diet in the UK and Scotland and highlighted some common problems, some similarities and some differences.

**Reference:**

➢ NICE Obesity in adults: Prevention & lifestyle weight management programmes 2016 (in development)

# 8. Physical Activity and Exercise

## Key Points

The risks of physical inactivity in relationship to CVD are similar to those associated with hypertension, high cholesterol and obesity.

In this chapter we look at physical activity. We will consider how exercise affects both cardiovascular and general health, the level of physical activity in the UK and the effects on mortality.

We will then consider in depth how you as GPs/Healthcare professionals can help your patients to increase their physical activity.

The aims of the chapter are to be able to promote the cardiovascular health of your patients by educating them about physical activity.

The objectives are as follows:
- To revise the risks of developing CVD from inadequate physical activity.
- To learn how exercise can improve cardiovascular health and how to talk to patients about this topic.

## 8.1 Physical Activity in England

- In England 24% men and 10% women undertake medium to vigorous activity for at least 30 minutes a day.
- 14% adults exercise regularly (EU average 9%).

- Over 10 years the percentage of men meeting physical activity requirements increased from 32% to 39% and women from 21% to 29%.
- In 2012 in England 67% men met recommended guidelines. 70% of highest incomes and 55% of lowest incomes. The highest levels of physical activity are undertaken in SE England 72% men and 61% women; the lowest in NW England.
- Percentage of boys and girls (age 5-15 years) achieving recommended levels fell between 2008 and 2012.
- Average distance walked or cycled per person per annum fell from 306 miles in 1975 to 221 miles in 2010.
- 15 million adults (57%) participate in sports at least once a month. Commonest sports are swimming, football and athletics.
- 62% men and 59% women consider themselves to be very or moderately active at work.
- There is a clear association between physical activity and BMI.

**References:**

➤ British Heart Foundation Physical Activity Statistics 2012 and 2015
➤ NHS Information Centre Statistics on Obesity, Physical Activity & Diet England 2013

### 8.1.1 Physical Activity in Scotland

- In 2010 45% men and 33% women in Scotland met Government recommendations for physical activity. Levels have slowly increased since the mid-1990s.
- Levels of physical activity in 2012 were the same in Scotland and England.
- In 2003 Scotland introduced a national physical strategy.
- In 2012 73% boys and 68% girls (age 2-15 years) met recommended levels of physical activity.
- By 2022 the target is 50% adults achieving minimum levels of activity.
- At present 2500 people in Scotland die prematurely each year from CHD due mainly to physical inactivity.
- Male life expectancy in the most disadvantaged areas is <70 years, in affluent areas it is 78 years.

**References:**

➢ British Heart Foundation CHD Statistics in Scotland 2012 and 2015
➢ Physical Activity Task Force (2003)


### 8.2 What Motivates People to Exercise?

Regular exercise is a multifactorial behaviour.


Factors which influence participation in and adherence to exercise include: Demographic and biological, psychological, cognitive and emotional, behavioural attributes and skills, social and cultural influences, physical environment and physical activity characteristics.

50% drop out within 6 months.

### 8.2.1 Why do People not take Exercise?

Lack of motivation.

Shortage of time.

Can't make regular commitment.

Affordability.

Lack of energy.

Physical or mental disability.

Hating exercise.

Exercise is Boring.

Self-conscious.

Don't see benefits.

Don't know how.

Impression that exercise hurts.

Perhaps you can think of additional reasons?

**Reference:**

> ➢ Kravitz L What motivates people to exercise IDEA Fitness Journal, Volume 8, Issue 1 2011

### 8.3 Physical Activity - Key Facts

Physical activity and exercise (or lack of them) are independent risk factors for many health conditions, as listed below.

People who take regular exercise have:

- up to a 35% lower risk of coronary heart disease and stroke.
- up to a 50% lower risk of type 2 diabetes.
- up to a 50% lower risk of colon cancer.
- up to a 20% lower risk of breast cancer.
- a 30% lower risk of early death.
- up to an 83% lower risk of osteoarthritis.
- up to a 68% lower risk of hip fracture.
- a 30% lower risk of falls (among older adults).
- up to a 30% lower risk of depression.
- up to a 30% lower risk of dementia.

**Reference:**

➤ NHS Choices Benefits of exercise 2013

## 8.4 Physical Activity and CVD

Now we are going to show how physical activity and exercise relates to CVD prevention.

We shall consider them separately from weight and diet, which have been covered in previous chapters.

Whilst one might believe that obesity arises from lack of physical activity or exercise, it has been difficult to show this scientifically, although there is some evidence that overweight and obese people do lead a more sedentary lifestyle. Whether or not this is causal or resulting from the weight problems remains unclear.

There is now emerging evidence that not only is physical activity and exercise important, but that episodes of sedentary behaviour can be damaging. Of course, to some extent people are not in control of how sedentary they are day to day, as this is influenced by their occupation, travel times, modes of life and so on. However, we should as health care practitioners be alerting our patients that the more sedentary time they spend, for example watching television or on the computer, the worse the health outcome. With an increased risk of all-cause and cardiovascular mortality, as well as diabetes.

Recommendations for type and degree of physical activity vary depending on an individual's age.

Survey studies have shown that in general British men, women and children do not engage in enough physical activity in their weekly routines.

**Reference:**
> British Nutrition Foundation Physical activity & Health 2007 Nutrition Bulletin 32. 314-363

## 8.5 Assessing Physical Activity

Physical activity is bodily movement produced by the contraction of muscles which substantially increases energy expenditure.

Exercise is planned, structured and repetitive bodily movements done to improve or maintain one or more component of physical fitness.

**Moderate intense activity** is activity which leads to becoming warm, breathing harder, with a faster heart beat but maintaining the ability to continue conversation.

**Vigorous intensity activity** is activity which leads to becoming much warmer, breathing much harder and heart beating more rapidly, making it difficult to continue a conversation.

The following are examples of moderate and vigorous activities:
Moderate = brisk walking, cycling.
Vigorous = jogging, swimming, football.

Ask your patient how often they do physical activity or exercise.

## 8.5.1 The Short Physical Activity Questionnaire

Helps you determine how much exercise your patient is doing.

As you can see, the questioning refers to how much physical activity your patient has undertaken within the last 7 days, categorising activity into mild, moderate and strenuous.

## 8.5.2 General Practice Physical Activity Questionnaire

Date...........................

Name.........................

1.  Please tell us the type and amount of physical activity involved in your work.

|   |   | Please mark one box only |
|---|---|---|
| a | I am not in employment (e.g. retired, retired for health reasons, unemployed, full-time carer etc.) | |
| b | I spend most of my time at work sitting (such as in an office) | |
| c | I spend most of my time at work standing or walking. However, my work does not require much intense physical effort (e.g. shop assistant, hairdresser, security guard, childminder, etc.) | |
| d | My work involves definite physical effort including handling of heavy objects and use of tools (e.g. plumber, electrician, carpenter, cleaner, hospital nurse, gardener, postal delivery workers etc.) | |
| e | My work involves vigorous physical activity including handling of very heavy objects (e.g. scaffolder, construction worker, refuse collector, etc.) | |

2.  During the _last week_, how many hours did you spend on each of the following activities? _Please answer whether you are in employment or not_

| | | None | Some but less than 1 hour | 1 hour but less than 3 hours | 3 hours or more |
|---|---|---|---|---|---|
| | | Please mark one box only on each row | | | |
| a | Physical exercise such as swimming, jogging, aerobics, football, tennis, gym workout etc. | | | | |
| b | Cycling, including cycling to work and during leisure time | | | | |
| c | Walking, including walking to work, shopping, for pleasure etc. | | | | |
| d | Housework/Childcare | | | | |
| e | Gardening/DIY | | | | |

3.  How would you describe your usual walking pace?  Please mark one box only.

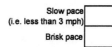

Slow pace (i.e. less than 3 mph) [ ]   Steady average pace [ ]

Brisk pace [ ]   Fast pace (i.e. over 4mph) [ ]

## Reference:

➢ Short Physical Activity Questionnaire NHS

https://www.gov.uk/government/...data/.../GPPAQ_-_guidance.pdf 2006

## 8.6 Guidelines for Physical Activity

The government in the UK is concerned about the rising obesity rates and increase in sedentary lifestyle of its inhabitants. As such, it has produced guidelines recommending activity levels per week.

- The United Kingdom Department of Health produced guidelines in 2011 recommending that adults (19-64 years of age) should aim for daily activity.
- This should add up weekly to at least 150 minutes of moderate intensive activity in episodes of 10 minutes or more, for example 30 minutes 5 times a week.
- Comparable benefits can be achieved by undertaking 75 minutes of vigorous intensity activity during a week.
- Adults should engage in muscle-strengthening activity on two occasions a week.
- Adults should minimise their time spent on sedentary activity.

**References:**

➢ The role of physical activity in counteracting obesity. Report on a joint WHO/ISBNPA technical consultation, Ljubljana, Slovenia. Copenhagen, WHO Regional Office for Europe 2012
➢ NICE Physical activity brief advice for adults in primary care May 2013

## 8.6.1 Recommendations for Physical Activity

Although guidelines state that the aim is to exercise moderately for 30 minutes 5 times a week, or intensively for 75 minutes a week, it should be recognised that starting off at this level from a sedentary lifestyle can also damage one's health. Impress upon your patient that levels of intensity and time taken to exercise need to be built up gradually. Exercise should be taken on a regular basis. They can take advice from GPs or from a sports professional, for example a personal trainer or trained exercise personnel.

People are more likely to do things they enjoy, and which they can easily fit into their weekly routine. Some people may prefer convenient, low-cost exercise such as jogging, brisk walking, or cycling, whilst others may benefit more from group activities, such as aerobic or dance classes, or team sports. Discuss with your patients which form of exercise they will enjoy doing, and what is realistic for them to integrate into their lives.

Although many domestic duties such as gardening and cleaning can be aerobically-demanding, carrying out these chores does not replace the need to undertake regular formal exercise. Formal exercise can ensure you reach and sustain the appropriate amount of aerobic and muscle-building challenges in a way that daily work duties cannot.

Using all that you have learnt so far, think of ways to converse with a patient about increasing the amount of physical activity they undertake in a week.

**Reference:**
- ➤ WHO Global recommendations on physical activity for health 2010

## 8.7 Motivating people to exercise

As with other life-style modifications, such as alcohol, tobacco and diet it is useful to apply the Prochaska/Di Clementi Transtheoretical model of change (See CVD Risk Factors and Primary Prevention chapter 3).

Pre-contemplation/Contemplation/Preparation/Action/Maintenance.

**Reference:**

➢ Kravitz L Exercise Motivation: What Starts and Keeps People Exercising?

https://www.unm.edu/~lkravitz/Article%20folder/ExerciseMot.pdf

## In Summary

In this chapter we have considered the modifiable CVD risk factor inadequate physical activity.

- We have outlined its relevance to the topic of cardiovascular health, and given some data about the nature and size of the problem in the UK and Scotland.

- Our aim has been to promote the cardiovascular health of your patients by educating them about the risks of inadequate physical activity and benefits of exercise.

- We have briefly outlined the topic of physical activity, and why it is important.

- We have suggested ways you can assess a patient's physical activity, and given some details on the UK's current recommendations, which you can choose to use as a framework for recommendations to your patients.

- We have demonstrated how exercise can improve cardiovascular health and how to talk to patients about the topic.

# 9. Stress

## Key Points

There is good evidence to show that stress increases a person's risk of CVD.

This chapter concentrates on the part stress may play in developing or aggravating CVD.

## Aim

- To recognise and diagnose stress in patients.
- To advise patients how to manage and reduce stress.

## 9.1 Stress and its Relationship to CVD

An extensive Whitehall Study in the UK among government employees found that those with the least control over their work had the highest rates of heart disease.

A meta-analysis of 13 European cohort studies (1985-2006), involving a combined 197,475 working adults from Finland, Sweden, Denmark, the Netherlands, Belgium, France, and England, found being stressed on the job was associated with a nearly 25% increased risk of CHD, and the association remained significant when adjusting for confounding factors.

In Australia, an expert group concluded that there is a strong and consistent link between depression, social isolation and lack of quality social support and heart disease. These factors were as risky to heart health as abnormal blood lipid levels, smoking and high blood pressure.

But the same group did not find a link between heart disease and chronic life events, job stress, Type A behaviour patterns, hostility, anxiety disorders or panic disorders.

However, other researchers have found a strong link between anxiety and heart disease.

Research is continuing in this area to define more clearly which kinds of stress are more likely to trigger CVD. Whatever the outcome may be, we already know that different types of stress tend to cluster together. When they do, the resultant risk for cardiac events is often substantially elevated.

**References:**
- Work Stress & Health: the Whitehall 11 study 2004
- Mika Kivimaki, Solja T Nyberg, G David Batty, Eleonor I Fransson, Katriina Heikkila. Lars Alfredsson, et al. "Job strain as a risk factor for coronary heart disease: a collaborative meta-analysis of individual participant data." Lancet, Sept. 14, 2012
- Bunker Stress & Coronary heart disease: psychosocial factors Med J Aust 2003, 178 (6): 272-6

### 9.2 Why do People get stressed?

Occupation such as prison service, police, social work, teaching, nursing and doctoring.

Long working hours.

Examinations and Interviews.

Separation or divorce of parents.

Illness or death of family member.

Changing schools or jobs.

Undertaking too many activities.

Loneliness.

Moving house.

Marriage.

Social problems with friends or family.

Peer pressure regarding smoking, drinking or drugs.

Bullying at school.

Friends moving away.

Not fitting into a group.

Changes in body weight or shape.

Low esteem.

Pre-menstrual.

Post traumatic, particularly in members of armed forces, fire services etc.

And many more causes.

**References:**

➢ American Psychological Association: "Mind/Body Health: Stress" Orth-Gomer, K. The Journal of the American Medical Association; 2000.

➢ www.webmd.com/balance/guide/causes-of-stress?page=2

## 9.3 Symptoms of Stress

Stress can affect how you feel, think, behave and how your body works. In fact, common signs of stress include sleeping problems, sweating, loss of appetite and difficulty concentrating.

You may feel anxious, irritable or low in self-esteem, and you may have racing thoughts, worry constantly or go over things in your head. You may notice that you lose your temper more easily, drink more or act unreasonably.

You may also experience headaches, muscle tension or pain, or dizziness.

With established coronary heart disease anxiety and stress, may bring on angina.

Some people try to cope with stress by smoking, drinking too much alcohol and overeating which increases their risk of CVD.

**Reference:**
 ➢ Health & Safety Executive Work-related stress signs & symptoms
   www.hse.gov.uk/stress/furtheradvice/signsandsymptoms.htm 2014

## 9.4 Assessing Stress

Questionnaires, such as the Holmes-Rahe Life Stress Inventory can be completed by the patient and may help to evaluate the severity of their stress and anxiety.

**Reference:**

> ➢ American Institute of Stress Holmes-Rahe Life Stress Inventory www.stress.org/holmes-rahe-stress-inventory

## 9.5 Stress Management

Lifestyle changes, such as balanced diet and regular physical activity will help you cope with stress.

Identifying and avoiding situations that make you feel stressed at home or at work, when possible, often helps reduce stress.

It important to learn how to relax. Yoga, tai chi, other relaxation techniques and techniques for managing stress engaged on a daily basis can help.

**Reference:**

> ➢ Smith M Stress Management Help Guide.org 2015
>
> http://www.helpguide.org/articles/stress/stress-management.htm

### 9.5.1 Aids to Relaxation

### 9.5.2 Relaxed Breathing

Practise deep breathing at a regular time and in a quiet place where you won't be disturbed. Loosen or remove any tight clothes you have on, such as shoes or jackets. Make yourself feel completely comfortable. Sit in a comfy chair which supports your head or lie on the floor or a bed. Place your arms on the chair arms, or flat on the floor or bed, a little bit away from the side of your body with the palms up. If you're lying down, stretch out your legs, keeping them hip-width apart or slightly wider. If you're sitting in a chair, don't cross your legs.

Good relaxation always starts with focusing on your breathing. The way to do it is to breathe in and out slowly and in a regular rhythm as this will help you to calm down.

- Fill up the whole of your lungs with air, without forcing. Imagine you're filling up a bottle, so that your lungs fill from the bottom.
- Breathe in through your nose and out through your mouth. Breathe in slowly and regularly counting from one to five.
- Then let the breath escape slowly, counting from one to five.
- Keep doing this until you feel calm. Breathe without pausing or holding your breath.
- Practise this relaxed breathing for three to five minutes, two to three times a day (or whenever you feel stressed).

### 9.5.3 Deep Muscle Relaxation

This technique takes around 20 minutes. It stretches different muscles in turn and then relaxes them, to release tension from the body and relax your mind.

Find a warm, quiet place with no distractions. Get completely comfortable, either sitting or lying down. Close your eyes and begin by focusing on your breathing; breathing slowly and deeply, as described above.

If you have pain in certain muscles, or if there are muscles that you find it difficult to focus on, spend more time on relaxing other parts.

You may want to play some soothing music to help relaxation. As with all relaxation techniques, deep muscle relaxation will require a bit of practise before you start feeling its benefits.

For each exercise, hold the stretch for a few seconds, then relax. Repeat it a couple of times. It's useful to keep to the same order as you work through the muscle groups:

- **Face**: push the eyebrows together, as though frowning, then release.
- **Neck**: gently tilt the head forwards, pushing chin down towards chest, then slowly lift again.
- **Shoulders**: pull them up towards the ears (shrug), then relax them down towards the feet.
- **Chest**: breathe slowly and deeply into the diaphragm (below your bottom rib) so that you're using the whole of the lungs. Then breathe slowly out, allowing the belly to deflate as all the air is exhaled.
- **Arms**: stretch the arms away from the body, reach, then relax.
- **Wrists and hands**: stretch the wrist by pulling the hand up towards you, and stretch out the fingers and thumbs, then relax.
- **Legs**: push the toes away from the body, then pull them towards body, then relax.

- Spend some time lying quietly after your relaxation with your eyes closed. When you feel ready, stretch and get up slowly.

**Reference:**

➢ NHS Choices Stress, anxiety & depression: Relaxation tips to relieve stress 2015

## In Summary

- How to understand the association between stress and CVD risk.
- How to recognise stress in your patient.
- How to evaluate significance of the stress.
- How to advise on self-management of stress.

## Management of Medical Problems

## 10. Hypertension

### Key Points

Raised blood pressure is a major risk factor for CVD and stroke.

The objectives of this chapter are shown below:

- To know how to diagnose and investigate Hypertension.
- To have a basic understanding of how to treat Hypertension.
- To know when to refer patients to specialists.
- To know where to access appropriate algorithms for reference and further learning.
- To use this knowledge to make management decisions.
- To discuss local factors that may affect these decisions.

In this chapter we review the investigation and treatment of Hypertension detailing appropriate management and treatment algorithms. We then consider a number of case vignettes. You can use these to discuss the management of patients with your colleagues. At the end of the chapter we will consider how as clinicians you can manage these conditions in your own practice.

### 10.1 Causes of Hypertension

In 90 to 95% of cases the cause is unknown. This is known as essential or **primary hypertension.**

Family history, possible genetic factors, increasing age, race - in North America the black population has an incidence twice that of the white, diet - increased salt consumption and low Potassium, Calcium and Magnesium and stress may all play a part in its development.

## Secondary Hypertension

In 5 to 10% of cases there are known defined causes. These include Diabetic nephropathy, Polycystic kidney disease, Glomerular kidney disease, Reno-vascular hypertension, Cushing's syndrome, Hyperaldosteronism, Phaeochromocytoma, Coarctation of the aorta, Lupus erythematosis. Prescription medications, for example, oral contraceptives, NSAIDs, decongestants, drugs used after organ transplants. Certain herbal remedies including ginseng and St John's Wort. Illegal drugs such as Cocaine, Amphetamine, crystal methamphetamine.

**Reference:**

➢ Bakris G Overview of Hypertension Merck Manual 2014

## 10.2 Isolated Systolic Hypertension

Increased vascular stiffness in those over 60 years causes increased pulse pressure, with increased risk of stroke. Blood pressure >140/<90 mm Hg.

Treatment is as for systolic & diastolic hypertension, but with low dose thiazide diuretics and slow/long-acting calcium antagonists.

**Reference:**

➢ van Zwietin P Drug treatment of isolated systolic hypertension Nephrol.Dial.Transplant (2001) 16 (6):1095-1097

## 10.3 Worldwide prevalence of Hypertension

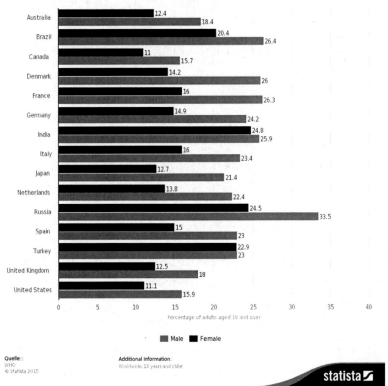

Prevalence of raised blood pressure in selected countries worldwide in 2014, by gender

**Reference:**

➢ http://www.statista.com/graphic/1/280143/prevalence-of-raised-blood-pressure-in-selected-countries-by-gender.jpg 2014

## 10.4 Hypertension in the UK

- There are 7 million people with diagnosed high blood pressure in the UK.

- In England 32% men and 29% women have high blood pressure.
- In Scotland 35% men and 30% women have high blood pressure.
- 5 million people in the UK have undiagnosed high blood pressure.
- Nearly 30% of adults in the UK have high blood pressure and up to 50% of these are not receiving treatment.

**Reference:**

➢ British Heart Foundation Coronary Heart disease Statistics 2012 and 2015

## 10.5 Hypertension - Measuring BP

Firstly let us highlight a number of considerations with regard to measuring blood pressure. As clinicians we have all been taught how to measure blood pressure.

However, devices for measuring blood pressure must be properly validated, maintained and regularly recalibrated according to the manufacturer's instructions.

If using an automated blood pressure monitoring device ensure that the device is validated and an appropriate cuff size for the person's arm is used.

When measuring blood pressure in the clinic or in the home standardise the environment and provide a relaxed, temperate setting, with the person quiet and seated and their arm outstretched and supported.

Palpate the radial or brachial pulse before measuring the blood pressure, since automated devices may not measure accurately if there is a pulse irregularity, such as atrial fibrillation. If a pulse irregularity is present, measure blood pressure manually, using direct auscultation over the brachial artery.

**Reference:**
> ➢ NICE Hypertension Guideline Page
> http://guidance.nice.org.uk/CG127

## 10.5.1 Hypertension - Diagnosis

**Clinic blood pressure**

As you know a raised blood pressure recorded at a single clinic visit should not be relied upon to make a diagnosis of hypertension. Take a second reading and if considerably different from the first, take a third reading. Record the lower of the last two readings as the clinic blood pressure.

**Confirming the diagnosis**

If the BP in the Clinic is above 140/90 it is recommended that the blood pressure is measured over a period of time in the person's own environment either using an ambulatory blood pressure recording device (ABPM) or by home blood pressure monitoring (HBPM) using an automated blood pressure machine.

## ABPM

If you are using an ambulatory recording device you should ensure that at least 2 valid measurements are made per hour during the person's normal waking hours. If this is not the case then you should either repeat the ambulatory recording or consider home blood pressure monitoring using an automated blood pressure machine.

If the ambulatory recording has been successful then you should average at least 14 measurements and use the average reading to confirm a diagnosis of hypertension.

## HBPM

If you are using home recording to confirm you diagnosis then each measurement should be taken twice, with the patient seated, and with 1 minute between measurements. The blood pressure should be recorded twice daily over at least 4 days, ideally for 7 days.

Discard the measurements taken on the first day and average the remaining measurements to confirm a diagnosis of hypertension.

Remember that an apparently raised blood pressure may be due to the white coat effect. The term 'white coat' comes from references to the white coats traditionally worn by doctors. The white coat effect means that your blood pressure is higher when it is taken in a medical setting than it is when taken at home.

**Further assessment**

While waiting for this confirmation of the diagnosis investigations to look for target organ damage can be carried out and a full assessment of cardiovascular risk factors can be made. Consider secondary causes of hypertension.

**Reference:**

> ➤ Ghuman N Role of Ambulatory and Home Blood Pressure Recording in clinical practice Curr Cardiol Rep. 2009 Nov; 11(6): 414–421.

## 10.6 Assessment of Target Organ Damage

It is important to assess whether there is any evidence of target organ damage.

Examine the retinal fundi for the presence of hypertensive retinopathy.

Test urine for the presence of protein and blood using a reagent dip strip and send a sample to the laboratory for albumin/creatinine ratio.

Take a blood sample to measure plasma glucose, electrolytes, creatinine, estimated glomerular filtration rate (eGFR), serum total cholesterol and HDL cholesterol.

Arrange for a 12- lead electrocardiograph to be performed.

**Reference:**

> Shlomai G Assessment of target organ damage in the evaluation and follow-up of hypertensive patients: where do we stand? J Clin Hypertens. 2013 Oct; 15(10):742-7

## 10.7 Degrees of Hypertension

Hypertension, in the past, has been classified as mild, moderate, severe and malignant, but the classification used here is the one adopted by the National Institute for Clinical Excellence and the British Hypertension Society in the UK. This classifies Hypertension as Stage 1, Stage 2, Severe and Accelerated. It employs both the clinic measurement and average BP. This classification of Hypertension is helpful because it directs the management.

**Stage 1 hypertension**

Clinic blood pressure is 140/90mm Hg or higher **and** subsequent ABPM daytime average or HBPM average blood pressure is 135/85mm Hg or higher.

**Stage 2 hypertension**

Clinic blood pressure is 160/100mm Hg or higher **and** subsequent ABPM daytime average or HBPM average blood pressure is 150/95mm Hg or higher.

**Severe hypertension**

Clinic systolic blood pressure is 180mm Hg or higher **or** clinic diastolic blood pressure is 110mm Hg or higher.

**Accelerated hypertension**

Clinic systolic blood pressure is 180mm Hg or higher **or** clinic diastolic blood pressure is 110mm Hg or higher and there are signs of papilloedema or retinal haemorrhage.

## 10.8 Management of Hypertension

**Stage 1 Hypertension**

In Stage 1 Hypertension the usual treatment would be to concentrate on lifestyle interventions, patient education and interventions to support adherence, to reduce BP and reduce cardiovascular risk, and to review annually.

However, if there is evidence of target organ damage or if the 10 year cardiovascular risk is greater than 20% then consider drug treatment in addition to these measures.

Young patients under 40 should be considered for referral to a specialist for investigation of secondary causes of hypertension and target- organ damage.

**Stage 2 Hypertension**

Patients with Stage 2 hypertension should be offered drug treatment in addition to lifestyle interventions, patient education and interventions to support adherence.

**Severe Hypertension**

Patients with Severe Hypertension should be offered drug treatment on the basis of clinic measurements alone without waiting for confirmation of the diagnosis by ambulatory BP monitoring or Home BP monitoring. These patients should also be offered lifestyle interventions, patient education and interventions to support adherence.

**Accelerated Hypertension**

Patients with accelerated hypertension or where you suspect a phaeochromocytoma should be referred to a specialist on the same day.

**Phaeochromocytoma** presents with anxiety or panic attacks, labile hypertension or postural hypotension, headache, palpitations, pallor or flushing and excessive sweating.

**Reference:**
  ➢ NICE Hypertension Clinical Management of primary hypertension in adults CG 127 2011

**10.9 Lifestyle Interventions**

Lifestyle advice should be offered initially and then periodically to all people undergoing assessment or treatment for hypertension.

Lifestyle interventions include advice and support on dietary change, increasing exercise, weight reduction, reducing alcohol consumption, reducing caffeine consumption, reducing Sodium intake and smoking cessation.

Use should be made of whatever aids are available such as written leaflets, audio-visual aids, computerised patient education, specific services within the healthcare system and patient support groups which promote lifestyle change. Relaxation therapies can reduce blood pressure and people may wish to try them.

In earlier chapters all these have been considered in greater detail.

**Reference:**

> ➤ Elhani S Lifestyle interventions in the management of hypertension: a survey based on the opinion of 105 practitioners Neth Heart J. 2009 Jan; 17(1): 9–12

## 10.10 Drug Treatment

Now let us turn to drug treatment in the UK.

**General principles:**

If drug treatment is to be successful the patient needs to adhere to their treatment and when planning treatment any measures that promote this should be encouraged. Try to use as few drugs as possible and try to use a once daily dosage regime.

Avoid combinations of drugs with similar modes of action. For example, do not combine an angiotensin-converting enzyme (ACE) inhibitor with an angiotensin 11 receptor blocker (ARB).

Isolated systolic hypertension ( if systolic blood pressure 160mm HG or higher) should be treated in the same way as patients with both systolic and diastolic hypertension.

Patients over 80 year old should be treated as younger patients. However, they are more at risk of side effects and drug interactions due to co-morbidities and polypharmacy, so caution needs to be employed.

An algorithm detailing drug treatment of hypertension can be found in NICE pathways 2016.

At each stage of treatment if the treatment appears to be ineffective it is important to consider patient non-adherence before adding additional drugs.

**Reference:**

> ➤ NICE pathways 2016

  pathways.nice.org.uk/pathways/hypertension

## 10.10.1 Patient Education and Adherence to Treatment
### Patient Education

- Help people to make informed choices by providing guidance and materials about the benefits of drugs and the unwanted side effects sometimes experienced.
- Tell people about patient organisations that have forums for sharing views and information.
- Offer an annual review of care to monitor blood pressure, provide people with support and discuss their lifestyle, symptoms and medication.

**Interventions to support adherence to treatment**

Only use interventions to overcome practical problems associated with non-adherence if a specific need is defined. Target the intervention to the need.

Interventions might include:

Encouraging self- monitoring their blood pressure. Suggesting self-recording their medicine-taking. Simplifying the dosage regime. Using alternative packaging for the medicine if the patient finds it difficult to open the medicine container, for example due to arthritic fingers. Using a multi-compartment medicine system.

Hypertension is often a symptomless condition and people may feel uncertain about the benefits of taking life-long medication especially if it has side effects, is difficult to take or is expensive. Education and support is needed in order to encourage patient adherence to advice and treatment.

**Reference:**
 ➢ Sandra van Dulmen Patient adherence to medical treatment: a review of reviews BMC Health Services Research 2007, 7:55

**10.10.2 Goals of Treatment and Monitoring**

**Monitoring Treatment**

When monitoring treatment generally use clinic blood pressure measurement. However if a patient appears to be susceptible to the white coat effect then consider Home BP monitoring or Ambulatory BP monitoring as a way of assessing response to treatment.

## Blood Pressure Targets

**Clinic blood pressure:** People aged under 80 years aim for BP lower than 140/90mm Hg. People aged over 80 years aim for BP lower than 150/90mm Hg.

**Daytime average ABPM or average HBPM blood pressure during waking hours:** People aged under 80 years aim for BP lower than 135/85mm Hg. People aged over 80 years aim for BP lower than 145/85 mm Hg.

There is no evidence for the optimal period between reviews of medication once a person's BP is controlled. However, it is recommended that a minimum of an annual face to face review of BP and medication is conducted.

**Reference:**
- ➤ NICE Hypertension Guideline Page
  http://guidance.nice.org.uk/CG127

## Case Vignettes

How would you manage each of the following two cases?

Discuss each case with a colleague and from the clinical features of the case construct a management plan for the patient. Then write down the reason why you have made these decisions.

## Case 1

A 40 year old man attends your surgery with a chest infection. He admits to smoking 40 cigarettes a day. On examination you find his BP to be 162/100. His HeartScore 10 year risk is 20%.

## Case 2

A 60 year old woman is found to have a persistently raised BP (average on home monitoring of 146/94). She admits to drinking 30 units of alcohol weekly. Her serum creatinine is 130 mmol/l (reference range 45-90) and her urinary albumin/creatinine ratio is raised.

### What can you do?

Consider, what are the local issues in the UK in relation to the management of hypertension and how these might be modified to ensure the best care for your patients?

Consider and discuss with a colleague how you would manage hypertension. Also consider the problems you may face in managing these patients and any practical solutions to these problems. Write these down.

### In Summary

In this chapter you have:

- Re-enforced your knowledge regarding diagnosis, investigation and management of Hypertension and reviewed when to refer patients to the specialists.

- Considered the application of this knowledge to clinical cases.
- Begun to consider local issues in the UK that might affect your ability to manage these patients.

# 11. Cholesterol

## Key Points

Raised levels of cholesterol are a major risk factor for CVD.

In this chapter we review the use of lipid lowering drugs in the primary prevention of CVD and detail appropriate management.

## Objectives:

The objectives of this chapter are shown below:

- To look at the incidence of raised cholesterol in the UK.
- To know when to use lipid lowering drugs for Primary prevention of Cardio-Vascular Disease.

### 11.1 The role of Lipids in the Development of CVD

Meat, poultry, eggs and dairy products are the main dietary sources of cholesterol and triglycerides.

Cholesterol and triglycerides are transported in the blood by lipoproteins to the liver. There they are metabolised to very low density lipids (VLDL) which are secreted into the plasma and converted initially to intermediate density lipids (IDL) and subsequently to low density lipids (LDL).

These can be deposited on the arterial intima forming atheromatous plaques. High density lipids (HDL) transport cholesterol to the liver where it is excreted into the intestine.

**Reference:**

> ➢ Blaton V The role of lipids and CHD: guidelines for diagnosis and treatment vol 14 2 International Federation of Clinical Chemistry and Laboratory Medicine (IFCC) 2003

## 11.2 Secondary Causes of Hyperlipidaemia

Nephrotic syndrome, hypothyroidism, biliary obstruction, pregnancy, myeloma, porphyria, steroids, obesity, diabetes mellitus, renal failure, excess ethanol intake, beta blockers, thiazide diuretics, isotretinoin, oral contraceptive pill, lipodystrophies, glycogen storage disease may all be associated with raised cholesterol levels.

## 11.3 National Prevalence of Raised Cholesterol Levels

In 2012 73% of the population of Bulgaria had raised cholesterol levels, whilst in Finland the proportion was 24%, with similar levels in USA, Australia, Canada, Thailand, Israel and the UK. In Lithuania, Romania, Ukraine, Hungary and Russia levels were high.

**Reference:**

> ➢ Global variation in the presence of elevated cholesterol according to National indices of economic development Circulation 2012; 125:1858-1869

## 11.3.1 Cholesterol in the UK

- In 2008 in the UK 22 million people had a raised total cholesterol level (population 60 million).
- In 2008 the percentage of the population of England with raised cholesterol showed regional variations of 54-64% in men and 56-68% in women.

**Reference:**

➢ Coronary Heart Disease Statistics 2012 176-180

## 11.4 Cholesterol Levels and CVD Risk

The rate of development of CVD relates to different levels of HDL-cholesterol. The higher the levels of HDL-cholesterol the lower the risk of CHD.

Optimal level of total cholesterol should be <5 mmol/l, of LDL cholesterol 3.0 mmol/l or less and of HDL-cholesterol >1.2 mmol/l in men and >1.0 mmol/l in women.

1% decrease in total cholesterol reduces CVD mortality by 2.5%.

**Reference:**

➢ Lipid modification: cardiovascular risk assessment and the modification of blood lipids for the primary and secondary prevention of cardiovascular disease NICE clinical guideline 181 2015

### 11.4.1 Familial Hyperlipidaemia

Autosomal dominant inheritance of FH gene. A raised total cholesterol level is present from birth. Prevalence is 1 in 500. There are approximately 110,000 carriers in UK. By the age of 50 years male carriers have a 50% risk of a CVD event and by age of 60 years female carriers have a 30% risk.

**Reference:**

➢ NICE guideline CG71 Familial hyperlipidaemia identification and management

## 11.4.2 Trans Fatty Acids

Trans fatty acids (TFA) are formed when oil is hydrogenated and is used industrially for frying and as an ingredient in processed foods. A diet high in TFA increases cholesterol levels. Intake of TFA can be reduced by avoiding products containing them, such as processed foods, biscuits, cakes and pastries and using vegetable oil for frying. The European Commission (EC) plans to limit permitted levels of TFA present in food and drinks.

**Reference:**

➢ Report from EC to European Parliament regarding trans fats in foods December 2015

http://ec.europa.eu/food/safety/docs/fs_labelling-nutrition_trans-fats-report_en.pdf

## 11.5 Pharmacological Treatment of Hypercholesterolaemia in Primary Prevention of CVD

The decision as to whether to prescribe a lipid lowering drug is based on an assessment of the patient's risk of CVD. This includes the use of risk scores such as Heart Score &/or QRISK2 to calculate the patient's 10 year risk of developing CVD and also clinical assessment of other patient factors that are not included in this assessment, such as patient preferences as well as other co-morbidities and drug treatments.

If a patient has severe hyperlipidaemia or you suspect from your patient's history that there may be a familial lipid disorder then you should consider further investigation and referral to a specialist.

Even if your decision is that drug treatment is appropriate for your patient it is very important to emphasise the necessity for lifestyle modification and explain that this pill does not remove the need to address these issues.

**If, using the risk assessment tool, the 10 year risk of CVD is shown to be less than 20%** then lifestyle modification should be advised and the risk assessed on an on-going basis. However, if risk is near the threshold, you should also consider the presence of other risk factors which may indicate that lipid lowering drug treatment may be appropriate. These include other chronic disease associated with increased risk e.g. Chronic Kidney Disease, Rheumatoid Arthritis, Systemic Lupus Erythematosus, mental Illness such as Schizophrenia.

**If the 10 year risk is 20% or more** then before considering starting lipid modifying drugs emphasise the importance of lifestyle modification and assess the patient's full lipid profile, BP, Fasting Blood Glucose, Renal function, Liver function (transaminases) and Thyroid Function (TSH).

NICE is considering recommending reducing the level at which statins should be started to a 10 year risk of 10%.

Offer Simvastatin 40mgm a day. If there are potential drug interactions or 40mgm is contraindicated change to Simvastatin 20mgm or Pravastatin 40mgm.

Statins are most effective if taken in the evening, but a proportion of patients experience insomnia. In which case they can take the medication with breakfast.

Grapefruit increases the plasma concentration of Simvastatin and patients should be advised to avoid it.

High dose statins, fibrates and anion exchange resins should not be routinely used for primary prevention.

There is no formal target for Total cholesterol or LDL-cholesterol in primary prevention and repeat lipid profile testing is not necessary. Review the drug therapy in line with good clinical practice, aiming to reduce risk. Measure liver function at 3 and 12 months, but not again unless clinically indicated.

If drugs that interfere with statin metabolism are introduced to treat other conditions then consider reducing or stopping statins (for example, Pravastatin concentrations are increased with concomitant Erythromycin and this is associated with increased risk of myopathy).

Among people without evidence of CVD treated prophylactically with statins mortality, major vascular events and revascularisation were reduced with no excess of adverse events.

In 2013 new guidelines were introduced in the USA, based on recommending statins only for the following groups:

i)   Individuals with clinical atherosclerotic CVD;

ii)  Individuals with LDL >190 mg/dl (4.9mmol/l) e.g. familial hypercholesterolaemia;

iii) Diabetics aged 40 - 75 years without clinical CVD and LDL 70-189 mg/dl (1.8-4.8mmol/l);

iv)  Non-diabetic individuals with no clinical CVD but LDL 70-189 mg/dl (1.8-4.8mmol/l) plus 10 year risk >7.5%.

**Reference:**

> Stone NJ, et al. 2013 ACC/AHA guideline on the treatment of blood cholesterol to reduce atherosclerotic cardiovascular risk in adults: A report of the American College of Cardiology & American Heart Association. J Am Coll Cardiol 2013

**11.5.1 Side Effects of Statins**

Serious side effects are rare but it is important that all patients started on a statin should be warned to seek medical advice if they develop muscle pain, muscle tenderness or muscle weakness as this may indicate the development of the rare severe myositis associated with statin treatment, rhabdomyolysis. Creatine Kinase levels should be measured in these patients.

Common side effects include nose bleeds, sore throat, non-allergic rhinitis, headache, nausea, constipation, diarrhoea, indigestion or flatulence, muscle and joint pain, hyperglycaemia.

Uncommon side effects include vomiting, loss of appetite or weight gain, insomnia or having nightmares, dizziness, peripheral neuropathy, memory problems, blurred vision, tinnitus, hepatitis, flu-like symptoms, pancreatitis, stomach pain, acne or an itchy red rash, feeling of tiredness or weakness.

Rare side effects (affecting 1 in 1000 people) include visual disturbances, bleeding or bruising easily, jaundice.

## 11.5.2 Cholesterol-Lowering Alternatives to Statins

If statins are not tolerated consider replacing statins with fibrates, anion-exchange resins, bile acid resins, Niacin (vitamin B3), Nicotinic acid, Colestyramine, Colestyrol or Ezetimibe.

Avoid the following foods: fatty cuts of meat and meat products, such as sausages and pies, butter, ghee and lard, cream, soured cream, creme fraiche and ice cream, cheese, particularly hard cheese, cakes and biscuits, chocolate, coconut oil, coconut cream and palm oil. The average man should have no more than 30g saturated fat a day and the average woman no more than 20g saturated fat a day. Eat a diet high in omega-3 fatty acids.

**References:**

- ➤ NICE Lipid Modificiation Guideline Page
  http://guidance.nice.org.uk/guidance/CG181
- ➤ Taylor Statins for the primary prevention of CVD Cochrane database 2014 Issue 1
- ➤ Guidelines for Management of Dyslipidaemias European Society of Cardiology 2011

### 11.5.3 Pharmacological Treatment of Hypercholesterolaemia in Secondary Prevention of CVD

All patients with clinical evidence of CVD should be offered a statin. This advice will be discussed in greater detail in chapter 13.

### In Summary

In this chapter you have:

- Learnt when to use pharmacological agents for primary prevention of CHD.
- Considered the application of this knowledge to clinical cases.

## 12. Diabetes Mellitus

### Key Points

People who develop diabetes are at increased risk of CVD and CVD is the leading cause of death among people with diabetes.

The objectives of this chapter are:

- To know how to diagnose and investigate Diabetes Mellitus (DM).
- To have a basic understanding of how to treat DM.
- To know where to access appropriate algorithms for reference and further learning.
- To know when and how to refer patients to specialists.
- To use his knowledge to make management decisions.
- To discuss local factors that may affect these decisions.

In this chapter we review the diagnosis, investigation and treatment of Diabetes Mellitus.

This will be followed by a presentation of appropriate management algorithms and where these can be accessed.

Then you should consider a number of case vignettes and use these to discuss with a colleague the management of patients presenting with these conditions.

Finally you should consider relevant factors in the UK and how as clinicians you can manage these conditions in your own practice.

## 12.1 The Causes of Diabetes

**Type 1 diabetes** occurs when autoimmune reactions destroy insulin-secreting pancreatic beta cells in the Islets of Langerhans. This may be triggered by viral and bacterial infections, chemical toxins in the diet, genetic factors or unknown causes.

**Type 2 diabetes** is associated with a positive family history, obesity, sedentary lifestyle, increasing age, unhealthy diet (processed foods, poor quality fats and low fibre content), pregnancy and metabolic syndrome.

**Metabolic syndrome** is characterised by obesity, insulin resistance, pro-inflammatory state (fibrinogen or plasminogen activator inhibitor-1 present in blood), dyslipidaemia (LDL raised, HDL low).

Poor glycaemic control in diabetics may increase LDL level.

**Reference:**
> http://www.niddk.nih.gov/health-information/health-topics/Diabetes/causes-diabetes/Pages/index.aspx

NIH Publication No. 14–5164 June 2014

## 12.2 Global Incidence of Diabetes

WHO estimates a worldwide incidence of 382 million diabetics.

### 12.2.1 Diabetes in the UK

- Over 3 million people in the UK are diabetic (7.4% of the population). 85-95% of these have Type 2 diabetes.

- By 2025 this will probably increase to 4.6 million.
- Possibly 500,000 cases are undiagnosed and 9.6 million at high risk of developing diabetes.
- Type 2 diabetes is increasingly common in children and adolescents.
- One in twenty people over 65 in the UK have diabetes.
- In 2010 there were 160,000 hospital admissions in the UK for diabetes.
- In 2014 the total annual bill for in-patient care for diabetics was £2 billion (11% of the total NHS expenditure).
- In Scotland 250,000 people (5% of the population) have diabetes; 217,000 of these have Type 2 diabetes.
- Since 2008 there has been a 25% increase in prevalence of diabetes in Scotland.

**References:**
➢ NHS Action for Diabetes 2013
➢ State of the Nation England Diabetes 2013 and 2015
➢ Scottish Diabetes Survey 2012 and 2015


### 12.3 Diagnostic Criteria for Diabetes

In 2006 WHO published diagnostic criteria for Diabetes. These are shown below:


Symptoms of diabetes - polyuria, polydipsia and unexplained weight loss plus fasting plasma glucose 7.0 mmol/l (126 mg/dl) or more or 2 hour plasma glucose (after 75g oral glucose load) 11.1 mmol/l (200mg/dl) or more or a random venous glucose concentration

11.1 mmol/l (200mg/dl) or more. You should note that in the absence of symptoms then a further plasma glucose measurement should be taken on another day.

In 2006 the WHO rejected the use of HbA1c as a diagnostic tool.

However, in 2011 they revised their advice and HbA1c is now used in addition to the previous criteria.

HbA1c 48 mmol/l (6.5%) or more is diagnostic of diabetes.

**Reference:**
  ➢ Diagnostic criteria for diabetes Diabetes UK 2015
    https://www.diabetes.org.uk

## 12.3.1 Situations where HbA1c is not appropriate for Diagnosis of Diabetes

- All children and young people.
- Patients of any age suspected of having Type 1 diabetes.
- Patients with symptoms of diabetes for less than 2 months.
- Patients at high diabetic risk who are acutely ill, such as those requiring hospital admission.
- Patients taking medication that may cause rapid glucose rise, for example steroids and antipsychotics.
- Patients with acute pancreatic damage, including pancreatic surgery.
- During pregnancy.

- Presence of genetic, haematological and illness-related factors that influence HbA1c and its measurement.

**Reference:**

➤ Southern Derbyshire Shared Care Pathology Guidelines Diagnosis of type 2 Diabetes Mellitus using HbA1c
  http://www.derbyhospitals.nhs.uk

### 12.3.2 Prediabetes

There are two other circumstances in which plasma glucose is considered to be abnormal while not diagnostic of Diabetes.

**Impaired Fasting Glycaemia and Impaired Glucose Tolerance**

These are not disease categories in themselves but indicate increased risk of developing diabetes and CVD.

The term **Impaired Glucose regulation (IGR)** has been introduced to classify individuals who have fasting plasma glucose values at the upper end of the normal range but below those diagnostic of diabetes and is demonstrated by IFG &/or IGT.

**Impaired Fasting glycaemia (IFG)**

This has been introduced to classify individuals who have fasting plasma glucose values at the upper end of the normal range but below those diagnostic of diabetes. Fasting plasma glucose 6.1 mmol/l or more but less than 7.0 mmol/l.

**Impaired Glucose Tolerance (IGT)**

This is a stage of impaired glucose regulation. Fasting glucose is less than 7.0 mmol/l and 2 hours after 75g oral glucose load value is 7.8 mmol/l or more but less than 11.1 mmol/l.

**Reference:**

➢ NICE guidelines PH38 2012
  https://www.nice.org.uk/guidance/ph38/chapter/glossary

## 12.4 Identifying Complications

Part of your role during diagnosis and annual monitoring is to identify complications of diabetes. Annual **Retinoscopy** will identify evidence of diabetic retinopathy and patients with established retinopathy should be referred to specialist care. Measurement of serum creatinine and urine albumin/creatinine ratio will enable detection of **Nephropathy**. Enquiry for symptoms of **autonomic neuropathy** and annual **examination of the feet** for circulatory and neuropathic damage should also be carried out. Look out for symptoms indicating **Peripheral vascular disease** or **Erectile dysfunction.**

**Reference:**

➢ Identifying & managing long-term complications diabetic pathway NICE 2015 http://pathways.nice.org.uk/pathways/diabetes

## 12.5 Management of Type 1 Diabetes

Here we remind you of the management in general of Type 1 diabetes, but we shall not be studying it in detail.

Diet and lifestyle advice.

Diabetes education.

Insulin.

Targets for treatment - HbA1c less than 7.5% (59 mmol/l)

**Reference:**

➤ NHS Choices Managing Type 1 Diabetes 2014

## 12.6 Management of Type 2 Diabetes

Once diagnosis has been made it is important that time be spent educating patients about diabetes and the need to modify their lifestyles. If there are no symptoms of diabetes and the plasma glucose is <15mmol/l then a trial of diet and lifestyle modification alone should be undertaken and the HbA1c measured in 3 months.

### 12.6.1 Diet and Lifestyle Advice

Now we detail the interventions that form part of the advice for newly diagnosed patients with type 2 diabetes.

**Dietary Advice**

- Provide individualised and ongoing nutritional advice from a healthcare professional with specific expertise and competencies in nutrition.
- Provide dietary advice in a form appropriate to the individual's needs, culture and beliefs, being sensitive to their willingness to change, and the effects on their quality of life.
- Emphasise advice on healthy balanced eating that is applicable to the general population when providing advice to people with Type 2 diabetes.

- Encourage high-fibre, low glycaemic index sources of carbohydrate in the diet, such as fruit, vegetables, whole grains and pulses, include low-fat dairy products and oily fish, and control the intake of foods containing saturated and trans fatty acids.
- Advise individuals that limited substitution of sucrose-containing foods for other carbohydrate in the meal plan is allowable, but that care should be taken to avoid excess energy intake.
- Discourage the use of foods marketed specifically for people with diabetes.
- Individualise recommendations for carbohydrate and meal patterns.
- Integrate dietary advice with a personalised diabetes management plan, including lifestyle modification, such as increasing physical activity and losing weight.

For those of you unfamiliar with the term **Glycaemic Index**. The Glycaemic Index (GI) is a ranking of carbohydrate containing foods based on their overall effect on blood glucose levels. Slowly absorbed foods have a low GI rating, whilst foods that are more quickly absorbed have a higher rating. Foods are given a GI number according to their effect on blood glucose levels. Glucose is used as a standard reference (GI 100) and other foods are measured against this. The effect on blood glucose levels over three hours, of a food portion (containing 50g of carbohydrate) is compared to the effect of 50g of glucose.

## Physical Activity

Advise patients to increase physical activity - any increase is beneficial.

## Weight Reduction

The target for people who are overweight is an initial body weight loss of 5–10%. Lesser degrees of weight loss may still be of benefit and larger degrees of weight loss in the longer term will have advantageous metabolic impact.

## Alcohol Intake

Individualise your recommendations. See chapter 6.

Patients can also be directed to patient organisations for peer support.

**References:**

➢ Lifestyle changes for Type 2 diabetes Diabetes.co.uk
  http://www.diabetes.co.uk/lifestyle-changes-for-type2-diabetes.html
➢ http://www.diabetes.org.uk/How_we_help/Local_support_groups/

### 12.6.2 Drug Therapy for Type 2 Diabetes

A management algorithm can be found in NICE Diabetes pathway 2015.

**Reference:**

➢ Blood-glucose-lowering therapy for type 2 diabetes
  http://pathways.nice.org.uk/pathways/diabetes/blood-glucose-lowering-therapy-for-type-2-diabetes 2015

## 12.7 Symptoms of Hypoglycaemia

Blood glucose less than 4 mmol/l (72 mg/dl).

The main symptoms associated with hypoglycaemia are:

Sweating.

Fatigue.

Feeling dizzy.

Symptoms of hypoglycaemia can also include:

Pallor.

Weakness.

Hunger.

A faster heart rate than usual.

Blurred vision.

Temporary loss of consciousness.

Confusion.

Convulsions.

Coma (extreme cases).

**Reference:**

> ➢ NHS Choices: Hypoglycaemia (low blood sugar) - Symptoms 2015

## 12.7.1 Management of Hypoglycaemia

**Immediate (self-administered)**

Sugary drink, fresh fruit, Dextrose tablets or sweets (all rapidly absorbed). Then few biscuits, cereal bar, fruit or sandwich.

Check blood glucose after 15-20 minutes.

**If unconscious**

Place in recovery position.

Glucagon injection adult dosage 0.25-2 mgm IV or 1-2 mgm IM.

If regains consciousness eat few biscuits, cereal bar or sandwich.

**References:**

➤ NHS Choices: Hypoglycaemic treatment 2015

➤ UK Hypoglycaemia Study Group (2007). Risk of hypoglycaemia in types 1 and 2 diabetes: effects of treatment modalities and their duration, Diabetologia 50: 1140-1147

## Case Vignettes

Let us consider 2 case vignettes.

Discuss each case with a colleague for about five minutes and from the clinical features of the case construct a management plan for the patient. Once you have decided on the management plan write down the reason why you have made these decisions.

**Case 1**

A 50 year old man presents with recurrent boils. He is otherwise well. He admits to smoking 30 cigarettes a day and drinking 40 units of alcohol a week (13 pints of strong lager / 1/3 bottle of whisky). On examination he has a BMI of 30. He is found to have a random blood sugar of 7mmol/l.

**Case 2**

A 55 year old woman has been diagnosed with type 2 Diabetes. She has been prescribed Metformin at the maximum dose. She has returned for review. Her HbA1c is 7.8.

## What can you do?

Consider, what are the issues in the UK in relation to the management of type 2 diabetes and how these might be modified to ensure the best care of your patients?

Please discuss with a colleague the opportunities in the UK for managing diabetes. Please also consider the problems you may face in managing these patients and consider any practical solutions to these problems. Write these down for future reference.

## In Summary

In this chapter we have:

- Reviewed the causes of diabetes.
- Reviewed the diagnosis and investigation of Diabetes Mellitus.
- Reviewed how to treat Diabetes Mellitus, including when to refer patients to a specialist.
- Used this knowledge to make management decisions.
- Begun to consider local issues in the UK that might affect your ability to manage these patients.

We hope that in this chapter you will have:

- Re-enforced your knowledge regarding diagnosis and management of Diabetes.
- Considered the application of this knowledge to clinical cases.

## Prevention Programmes

## 13. Secondary and Tertiary Prevention of Clinical CVD

### Key Points

Prevention of further disease in patients with existing CVD.

**Aims**

The aims of this chapter are:

- To know how to prevent further disease in patients with existing CVD.
- To know when and how to initiate preventive treatments, such as statins, anti-platelet drugs, beta-blockers, ACE inhibitors in patients with existing CVD.
- To know how to monitor patients and evaluate efficacy of preventive measures.
- To know when to refer to specialists.
- To understand principles of rehabilitation.

In this chapter we are mainly concerned with prevention in patients who already have diagnosed CVD.

We consider the need to continue to encourage lifestyle interventions and cardiac rehabilitation, medically manage specific risk factors and medical conditions that increase the patients' risk of CVD and consider specific preventive pharmacological interventions.

That is the basis of secondary and tertiary prevention. Working definitions of secondary and tertiary prevention are shown below.

### 13.1 Definitions of Secondary & Tertiary Prevention of CVD

**Secondary prevention** is the prevention of further episodes of symptomatic disease in patients who already have the disease.

**Tertiary prevention** is the prevention of deterioration in patients who have ongoing symptomatic disease.

**Reference:**

> The stages of prevention AFMC Primer on Population Health Part 1 Chapter 4

### 13.2 Lifestyle Interventions
### 13.2.1 Risk Factors

In patients who have established cardio-vascular disease it is important to identify lifestyle risk factors such as Smoking, Alcohol, Diet, Exercise, Obesity, Stress. Patients who have lifestyle related risk factors should be advised on the importance of addressing these and given help in doing this. The management of these has been covered in earlier chapters and will be repeated in this chapter.

### 13.2.2 Medical Interventions for Specific Risk Factors

In addition to managing lifestyle risk factors it is important to **optimise treatment for hypertension and diabetes** in patients who have these conditions by reviewing their management and ensuring that blood pressure and glycaemic control are optimal. We are not covering this in this chapter as earlier chapters have dealt with it. Also in addition to dietary interventions to reduce cholesterol the pharmacological treatment of raised cholesterol levels needs to be considered.

**Reference:**

➢ NICE Commissioning Guides

  https://www.nice.org.uk/guidance/cmg45/chapter/44-medical-interventions 2012

### 13.2.3 Cholesterol Modification

All patients with clinical evidence of CVD should be offered a statin. This recommendation is based on a meta-analysis of 14 studies carried out by the UK National Institute for Health and Clinical Excellence. This demonstrated that treatment with statins was associated with a reduction in all-cause mortality, CVD mortality, CHD mortality, fatal myocardial Infarct, unstable angina, hospitalisation for unstable angina, non-fatal stroke, new or worse intermittent claudication and coronary revascularisation.

When you initiate treatment baseline blood tests should be carried out (Fasting total cholesterol, LDL-cholesterol, HDL-cholesterol and triglycerides. Fasting blood glucose. Renal function, liver function, thyroid function). If any cause of secondary dyslipidaemia (such as hypothyroidism) is found, this should be treated.

The usual starting dose of Simvastatin is 40mg. Patients whose liver transaminases are raised can be prescribed statins so long as their transaminases are not greater than 3 times the upper limit of normal. All patients should be advised to seek advice if they develop muscle pain, tenderness or weakness. Their creatine kinase level should be measured.

**Reference:**

> NICE clinical guideline - Lipid Modification CG 181 2014

### 13.2.4 Follow-Up

The aim of treatment with statins is to reduce total cholesterol to less than 4mmol/l or LDL-cholesterol to less than 2mmol/l. However, less than 50% of patients will achieve this. If this is not achieved consider using higher doses of a statin. For example, Simvastatin 80 mgm daily if total cholesterol is more than 4 mmol/l or LDL-cholesterol more than 2 mmol/l.

Monitor liver function at 3 months and 1 year. If normal then there is no need for further monitoring unless clinically indicated.

If a patient develops symptoms or signs of a peripheral neuropathy that are not explained by another condition, for example diabetes, then stop the statin and refer to a specialist.

If statins are not tolerated then consider other pharmacological agents, such as Fibrates, Nicotinic acid, Anion exchange resins, Ezetimibe.

## 13.3 Patients presenting with Acute Coronary Syndrome (ACS)

Patients who present with an acute coronary syndrome - myocardial infarct, unstable angina, non-ST elevation myocardial infarct (NSTEMI), should be offered high dose statins, such as Simvastatin 80 mgm daily without waiting for the results of baseline blood tests. Their fasting lipids should be measured 3 months after starting treatment and monitored as above.

**Reference:**

> National Institute for Clinical Excellence. Myocardial infarction-Secondary prevention CG172 2013

## 13.3.1 Medical Interventions for ACS to Reduce Risks of Further Episodes of CVD

Research has indicated that certain pharmacological interventions which are not specifically aimed at risk factors can reduce patients' risk of further cardiovascular events following an acute coronary event. Patients who present with an acute coronary syndrome or who have a history of a proven myocardial infarction should be offered treatment with Angiotensin Converting Enzyme (ACE) Inhibitors, anti-platelet drugs and/or beta-blockers.

### ACE Inhibitors

A meta analysis of 18 randomised controlled trials in unselected patients immediately following an acute myocardial infarct (MI) found that ACE inhibitor treatment improved survival compared with placebo. Patients who have had a MI should have their left ventricular function assessed.

Renal function, electrolytes and BP should be measured before starting a patient on an ACE inhibitor or an Angiotensin 11 Receptor Blocker (ARB). These should be re-assessed 2 weeks after starting treatment.

All patients should be offered an ACE inhibitor early and the dose titrated up to the maximum tolerated dose. This should be continued indefinitely in patients with preserved Left Ventricular function or Left Ventricular Systolic Dysfunction (LVSD), whether or not they have heart failure symptoms.

If the patient is intolerant or allergic to an ACE inhibitor then use an (ARB).

Renal function, electrolytes and BP should be monitored after each dose increase. Renal function should be monitored frequently if the patient is at increased risk of a deterioration in renal function.

**Reference:**

➢ Saha SA Tissue ACE inhibitors for secondary prevention of cardiovascular disease in patients with preserved left ventricular function: a pooled meta-analysis of randomized placebo-controlled trials J Cardiovasc Pharmacol Ther 2007 Sep; 12(3):192-204

## Antiplatelet drugs

Offer Aspirin 75mg daily to all patients unless patient has Aspirin hypersensitivity. Aspirin should be continued indefinitely.

In patients with a history of Aspirin hypersensitivity offer Clopidogrel 75mg daily (otherwise do not use Clopidogrel alone).

In patient with a history of dyspepsia consider adding a proton pump inhibitor (PPI). If there is a history of aspirin- induced ulcer bleeding and the ulcer has healed and the patient is H. pylori negative consider aspirin plus full dose PPI.

In patients who have had an ST segment elevation myocardial infarct (STEMI) offer Clopidogrel in addition to Aspirin for 4 weeks

In patients who have had a non ST segment elevation acute coronary syndrome (NSTEMI-ACS) offer Aspirin and Clopidogrel or Ticagrelor for 12 months if there is a moderate to high risk of MI or death. After this period continue with Aspirin alone.

The risk of MI or death in patients with NSTEMI-ACS can be determined from clinical signs and symptoms plus clinical investigations indicating on-going myocardial ischaemia and/or raised blood levels of markers of cardiac cell damage, such as troponin.

**Reference**:

➢ Updates in antiplatelet agents used in cardiovascular diseases J Cardiovasc Pharmacol Ther. 2013 Nov; 18(6):514-2

**Beta-blockers**

A meta analysis of 31 long term randomised controlled trials (6 weeks to 48 months) found that treatment with beta- blockers in patients after acute MI reduced the odds of death by 23% compared with placebo.

Once a patient is clinically stable after MI offer all patients a beta-blocker and increase the dose to the maximum tolerated dose and continue indefinitely. However, consider comorbidities such as bradyarrhythmias, hypotension and chronic obstructive airways disease which may make the patient unsuitable for a beta-blocker therapy. If left ventricular systolic dysfunction (LSVD) is present use a beta-blocker licensed for the treatment of heart failure e.g. Bisoprolol, Carvedilol or Nebivolol.

If it is longer than 12 months since the MI and there is no evidence of LVSD, even if the patient is asymptomatic, offer a beta-blocker. However, if left ventricular function is preserved, with no symptoms, do not routinely offer treatment with a beta-blocker.

**Reference:**

➤ Freemantle, N., Cleland, J., Young, P. et al Beta-blockade after myocardial infarction: systematic review and meta regression analysis. BMJ 1999; 318:1730-1737

**Long-term Management**

Patient follow up after a coronary event needs to consider the following areas:

## Identification of deterioration in CVD

Clearly patients need to be monitored to identify whether there has been a deterioration in the patients cardiovascular status. Identification of new ischaemic symptoms, such as angina or deteriorating cardiac function resulting in heart failure, is important so that measures can be taken to improve the patient's condition by modifying their drug therapy and referring them to a specialist when needed.

## Support of lifestyle interventions

Research has shown that only about 30% of patients who need lifestyle modification for the long term-management of their conditions adhere to it. An important function of following up such patients is to reinforce the need for lifestyle change.

## Medical management of risk

The medical management of risk includes monitoring the management of risk factors such as diabetes and hypertension. It also includes the monitoring of pharmacological interventions for side effects e.g. deterioration in renal function with ACE inhibitors. Similarly, as in the case of lifestyle interventions, adherence to medication may be an issue and active monitoring of this and supportive measures to encourage adherence are an important aspect of follow up.

**Reference:**

➤ National Clinical Guideline Centre (2013) Post myocardial infarction: secondary prevention in primary and secondary care for patients following a myocardial infarction (full guideline).

## 13.4 Cardiac Rehabilitation

- Group based cardiac rehabilitation programmes reduce cardiovascular morbidity and mortality by reducing recurrent events, improving risk factors, assisting pharmacotherapy adherence and enhancing quality of life.
- Although cardiac rehabilitation has been proven to be beneficial, uptake has been suboptimal (40% uptake among heart attack survivors in the UK).
- When cardiac rehabilitation services are planned, the needs of the particular local community should be taken into account, including health and social factors and deprivation. Services should be culturally sensitive.
- The physical components should be adapted to meet the needs of older patients and those with significant comorbidities.
- Patients should be offered mixed-sex or single-sex classes.
- It is important for patients' health beliefs and basic level of health literacy to be established before lifestyle advice is offered.
- All healthcare professionals who come into contact with post-MI patients, including senior medical staff, should promote cardiac rehabilitation services.

**Phase 1: the initial stage following MI or cardiac event**

Assessment of a patient's physical/psychological condition. Assessment of risk factors. Initial mobilisation. Plan for discharge from hospital.

**Phase 2: the post-discharge stage**

The early discharge period is the time at which the patient is the most vulnerable and psychological distress at this stage is a predictor of poor outcome.

**Phase 3: structured exercise and rehabilitation**

Graded exercise is a vital component of cardiac rehabilitation. Aerobic low-to-moderate intensity exercise will be suitable for most patients who have been assessed as low-to-moderate risk.

**Phase 4: long-term maintenance**

In order to be effective, physical activity and changes in lifestyle need to be maintained for the long-term. This necessitates long-term monitoring.

**References:**

➢ NICE Commissioning a cardiac rehabilitation service CMG40 2014

➢ Piepoli Secondary prevention through cardiac rehabilitation Eur. J. Cardiovasc Prev Rehabil 2010. 17:1-17

## Case Vignettes

Spend five minutes discussing each of the following cases with a colleague and construct & write down a management plan for the patient.

## Case 1

A 50 year old man presents to you with a history that he was admitted to hospital with a myocardial infarct in another city 6 months ago. He was given some medication when he was discharged, but has not taken any medication since these finished as he has felt well and did not think he needed them.

## Case 2

A 60 year old woman who had a myocardial infarct 2 years ago and takes Aspirin 75 mgm daily, Simvastatin 40 mgm daily, Ramipril 2.5 mgm daily and Atenolol 25 mgm daily. She consults complaining of a cough for 2 weeks. On further questioning she admits that she is still smoking 20 cigarettes a day. On examination she has signs of consolidation in the upper lobe of her right lung. She is allergic to Penicillin.

## In Summary

In this chapter you should have learnt:

- How to prevent further disease in patients with existing CVD.
- The importance of changing their behaviour and continuing lifestyle modification.
- When and how to initiate preventive treatments, such as statins, anti-platelet drugs, beta-blockers, ACE Inhibitors.

- How to monitor patients and evaluate efficacy of preventative measures.
- When to refer patients to specialists.
- The value of cardiac rehabilitation.

# 14. Implementing Change: Planning a Preventive Cardiology Programme

## Key Points

Planning a preventive cardiology programme by Implementation of changes in professional behaviour and practice in relevant healthcare settings.

In the preceding chapters we have shown you how to recognise patients at risk of developing CVD and how to advise and assist them by applying appropriate measures to reduce their individual risk. The aim of this chapter is to consider how changes in professional behaviour and practice can be practically implemented in relevant healthcare settings when planning a preventive cardiology programme.

## Objectives:

- To confirm the need for establishing CVD prevention programmes.
- To identify potential barriers to implementing necessary changes.
- To generate ideas to help overcome the barriers.
- To take away a plan to promote local programme implementation.
- To consider methods of monitoring and evaluating programme performance.

We shall cover:

- Cost-effectiveness of prevention.
- Burden of CVD.
- Potential for Change.
- Barriers to preventive approach.
- Prevention strategies.
- Population based and high risk approach.

We then ask you to spend some time at the end of the chapter discussing with a colleague how the ideas we presented relate to your local circumstances and how some of the changes we proposed could be implemented in your practice.

It might be useful just to agree some basic assumptions which have been covered in previous chapters.

## 14.1 Basic Assumptions

CVD is a major healthcare problem in the UK and worldwide resulting in serious human and economic costs.

There is great potential for prevention at national, regional and local levels.

Health promotion and disease prevention should receive greater emphasis in the training of all health professionals.

Greater attention is needed to identify individuals at risk.

Greater priority should be given to risk factor management.

### 14.1.1 Recapitulation

- Most CVD is due to reduced blood flow to the heart, brain or body caused by atheroma or thrombosis. It is increasingly common after the age of 60 but rare below the age of 30.
- The main types of CVD are: coronary heart disease (CHD), stroke and peripheral vascular disease (PVD).
- Morbidity and mortality in the UK has significantly improved, but there is still room for further improvement.
- The major modifiable risk factors linked to CVD are: smoking/tobacco use, poor diet, raised blood cholesterol, high blood pressure, insufficient physical activity, overweight/obesity, diabetes, psychosocial stress (linked to people's inability to influence the potentially stressful environments in which they live) and excessive alcohol consumption.
- Many CVD risk factors are also associated with other health-related conditions including some common cancers, chronic respiratory disease, obesity, diabetes, kidney disease and mental health. A positive approach to cardiovascular prevention is therefore likely to also help prevent some of these other health problems.

The focus in this chapter is on regional and local programmes led by healthcare professionals. However, it must be remembered that these measures should ideally be in the context of national policies, which may include major areas such as education, taxation, agriculture, food regulation, building and transport. Policies in these areas may have a powerful impact on people's lifestyle and health. They also impact on climate change and sustainable development which, in turn, can affect health.

### 14.1.2 Modifiable Risk Factors

Smoking, Alcohol, Diet, Weight, Physical Activity, Blood Pressure, Lipids, Diabetes, Stress are all potentially modifiable.

So we know what people need to do, namely, modify risk factors. The main questions for preventive cardiology are:

- *How do we educate people about risk, both the general population and health professionals?*
- *How do we identify those at higher risk?*
- *How do we help those people to reduce their risks?*

The answers may seem simple in theory and yet in much of the world the problem is not being effectively tackled.

Why might this be?

### 14.2 The Burden of CVD in the UK

- In 2012 CVD caused 28% of all deaths.
- In 2012 in the UK 26% of premature deaths in men aged <75 years were due to CVD.
- In 2012 74,000 people died from CHD.

- In 2012 >1.6 million CVD related episodes were admitted to NHS hospitals.
- It was estimated that in 2015 there are 7 million people living with CVD in the UK (3.5 million men and 3.5 million women).

**Reference:**
 ➢ British Heart Foundation CVD Statistics UK Fact Sheet 2016

## 14.3 The Impact of CVD in the UK

- In 2012/13 >£6.8 billion was spent on treating CVD in England.
- Total CVD costs have risen from £5.3 billion in 2003/4. CVD direct health costs in 2009 were £8.6 million, productivity loss from deaths £4 million and morbidity £2.4 million. The total costs equated to 6% of total healthcare expenditure. This rose to 7.2% in 2011, but still remained a significantly lower percentage than that of the United States and most Western European countries.
- By 2014 total cost of CVD in the UK, including indirect costs from premature death and disability, had risen to £15 billion annually.
- Mortality rates from CVD in the UK are 50% higher in the most deprived regions than in the least deprived.
- Death rates from CHD are higher in the lower social classes than in the higher social classes.

**References:**
 ➢ Prevention of CVD: Costing report NICE June 2012
 ➢ British Heart Foundation CD Statistics - UK Fact sheet 2015

## 14.4 Health Needs Assessment

The purpose of health needs assessment in healthcare is to gather information required to bring about change and benefits to health of the population.

Information can be gathered from a variety of sources by Rapid participatory appeal, such as community assessment. From existing documents, interviews and direct observation. By Postal surveys. From Local statistics, such as hospital-based morbidity. From Practice held information.

**References:**

➢ Stevens Needs Assessment: from theory to practice BMJ 1998; 316:1448

➢ Murray Practice based health needs assessment. Use of 4 methods in a small neighbourhood BMJ 1995; 310:1443

➢ NICE Health Assessment guidance 2005

## 14.5 CVD in hard to reach Population

The aged, disabled, homeless, prisoners, drug addicts and migrants must not be forgotten and require appropriately designed measures to trace and assist.

Greater Manchester Public Health Network takes prevention to such individuals in a double-decker bus.

North West Midlands has devised a regional development plan to cope with the problem in their region.

**References:**

➢ Bonevski B Reaching the hard-to-reach: a systematic review of strategies for improving health and medical research with socially disadvantaged groups BMC Medical Research Methodology 2014, 14:42

➢ First Stop Health Bus www.gmphnetwork.org.uk

➢ Regional Development of a Population based collaboration CVD Prevention Strategy. The experience of NHS West Midlands NICE CVD guidance expert testimony paper 5 2007

### 14.6 The Potential for Change

Evidence from developed and developing countries has shown that individuals with increased risk of CVD can reduce their risk of cardiovascular morbidity and mortality by stopping smoking, changing their diet, reducing alcohol intake, engaging in physical activity, achieving a healthy body weight and controlling their blood pressure, cholesterol and diabetes.

**Reference:**

➢ Graham I, Atar D, Borch-Johnsen K, et al. European guidelines on cardiovascular disease prevention in clinical practice: executive summary. Fourth Joint Task Force of the European Society of Cardiology and Other Societies on Cardiovascular Disease Prevention in Clinical Practice (Constituted by representatives of nine societies and by invited experts). Eur Heart J 2007; 28:2375–414

### 14.7 Barriers to Achieving CVD Reduction

You will see listed below some of the barriers:

- Limited recognition of size of CVD problem.
- Health promotion and disease prevention not taken as seriously as treatment and cure.
- Stroke and CVD considered as diseases for specialists to manage.
- Health care costs are increasing and resources are decreasing.
- Established cultural concepts.

**Reference:**

➤ Benjamin E et al Magnitude of the Prevention problem: opportunities & challenges J Am Coll Cardiol 202; 40(4):588-603 2002

**14.8 Barriers to Implementation of Preventive Services**

**Healthcare systems**

Acute care priority

Lack of resources

Lack of training

Lack of systems

Time and economic constraints

Lack of policies and standards

**Community**

Lack of knowledge

Lack of motivation

Cultural factors

Social factors

The fundamental contribution of lifestyle behaviors to the prevention and reduction of risk factors, and the high prevalence of risk factors in most population groups means that a **public health approach** to preventing CVD is essential. Health education is essential in the general population. **Legislation** to reduce alcohol and tobacco availability and usage also plays a very significant part in reducing CVD risk, for example smoking bans in public places.

But **we must also ensure that educational programmes for doctors, nurses and other health professionals give greater importance to prevention**. The emphasis in medical schools of many countries is still on diagnosing and treating acute illness. Students, in many instances, receive limited education in health promotion, disease prevention and the management of chronic conditions. Cardiologists, in particular, often view their role as managing the acute event. They frequently defer long-term prevention issues to primary care providers. The lack of specialist attention reinforces the perception on the part of primary care providers and patients that the treatment of chronic risk factors and lifestyle modification are discretionary practices.

Primary care physicians may feel overwhelmed by the question of how to prioritize risk factor reduction in a realistic and cost-effective manner. Health care providers need to understand and be able to communicate what the anticipated absolute benefit of a given risk-factor reduction strategy is in a specific patient. They must also be skilled in techniques for enhancing adherence to medication and lifestyle changes. Although probably all medical schools now include communication skills in their curricula, these skills may not always be reinforced in postgraduate training and continuing medical education programmes.

**Reference:**

> Cornuz J Physicians' attitudes towards prevention: importance of intervention-specific barriers and physicians' health habits Family Practice (2000) 17 (6):535-540

### 14.9 Developing Prevention Strategies

The development of many strategies for the prevention of CVD present an important policy question: *Do the benefits of these programmes and interventions justify the investment in them?* Preventive strategies may provide attractive opportunities to avoid or defer disease and disability, but they may have substantial costs and must often be applied to many individuals in order to reach the few in the group who will benefit the most. Whether and how limited health care resources should be allocated to these activities is therefore an important question for health care policy makers and practitioners.

Fundamental questions such as: *Do the benefits of these programmes justify the investment? How much of our limited health care resources should be allocated to these activities? Will programmes cover the majority who are at risk? Who will benefit the most? What are the best approaches?* must be asked before embarking on any new strategy.

### 14.9.1 Cost Effective Strategies in CVD Prevention

Discussion continues regarding the cost-effectiveness of preventive measures.

In some instances the measures may only benefit a very small proportion of the population and can be more expensive than treating the developed condition.

However, there is general agreement that targeting those at high risk increases the cost-effectiveness. Certain measures, in particular tobacco and alcohol screening and counselling, reduction of hypertension by dietary salt restriction, weight loss and exercise, daily low dose aspirin in secondary CVD prevention, cholesterol screening and statin use are generally recognised to be cost-effective.

Any intervention that achieved even a modest population-wide reduction in any major cardiovascular risk factor would produce a net cost saving to the NHS, as well as improving health.

A programme across the entire population of England and Wales (about 50 million people) that reduced cardiovascular events by just 1% would result in savings to the health service worth at least £30m (€34m, $48m) a year compared with no additional intervention.

Reducing mean cholesterol concentrations or blood pressure levels in the population by 5% would result in annual savings worth at least £80m to £100m. Measures to reduce dietary salt intake by 3 g/day (current mean intake approximately 8.5 g/day) would prevent approximately 30,000 cardiovascular events, with savings worth at least £40m a year. Reducing intake of industrial trans fatty acid from present proportion of 0.8% to 0.5% of total energy content might gain around 570,000 life years and generate NHS savings worth at least £230m a year.

**References:**

- Cohen J. Does Preventive Care save money? N Eng J Med 2008,358.661-663
- Alcohol & tobacco screening and counselling are cost-effective The Synthesis Project Policy Brief No 18 Sep 2009 Robert Wood Johnson Foundation
- Barton Effectiveness & cost effectiveness of CVD prevention in whole population: modelling study BMJ 2011; 343:d4044

### 14.9.2 Three Levels of Prevention

When considering any prevention programme it is helpful to think in terms of three levels of prevention which should be addressed - as shown here. (Do not confuse these levels with primary, secondary and tertiary levels of prevention of clinical disease discussed in the previous chapter).

**Primary prevention** aims to prevent risk factors before they have started, for example health education in schools and advising all patients about benefits of healthy lifestyle.

**Secondary prevention** aims to detect and control risk factors, for example detecting and managing high blood pressure.

**Tertiary prevention** aims to manage established disease, for example treating patients who have already had MI or stroke to reduce complications, recurrence and further deterioration.

Some literature also refers to **primordial (or primal) prevention** which describes measures taken to ensure foetal well-being and prevent any long-term health consequences from gestational history and/or disease.

The term **quaternary prevention is** also sometimes used to describe measures to reduce risks of unnecessary or excessive interventions in the health system.

Any preventive programme needs to address all these levels in order to succeed.

**Reference:**
> What researchers mean by primary secondary & tertiary prevention At Work, Issue 80, Spring 2015: Institute for Work & Health, Toronto

**Two questions:**
*What are we currently doing to implement cardiovascular prevention in the UK?*
*What more can we aim to do and how?*

So at this point we would like you to discuss with colleagues what approaches you are aware are taking place in the UK and in your own local practices and clinics.

### 14.9.3 Strategies for Prevention

Two complementary strategies that are usually advocated for primary prevention are the 'population approach' and high-risk approach'.

In practice both approaches should be introduced to achieve maximal results.

**Reference:**

> ➤ NICE Services for prevention of CVD CMG45 2012

### 14.10 Population Based Approach

The population strategy aims to reduce the burden of disease in the whole community while conferring small benefits to each individual. Community wide interventions, such as smoke free areas and restrictions on advertising and sale of alcohol and tobacco, seek to modify behaviours and thereby influence the distribution of risk factors in the population. Even modest changes in risk factors are expected to contribute to a substantial reduction in the cumulative population risk of CVD because of the large number of people affected. There are small benefits to each individual.

The aim is to reduce morbidity and mortality from CVD by 2% per annum.

The population approach clearly requires support at a **public health and legislative level.**

- Culturally and linguistically appropriate and effective community health promotion and disease prevention programmes should be encouraged and made available. If they already exist they should be strengthened and integrated with the formal health care sector.
- CVD prevention should be integrated within primary AND secondary health care.
- Cardiovascular health education should be integrated with other health promotion initiatives, such as cancer and COPD reduction.
- Lifestyle advice should center on smoking cessation, reduced alcohol consumption, weight control, a heart-healthy diet, physical activity and stress management.
- Cardiovascular health promotion should be part of the national media strategy.
- Cardiovascular health should be addressed in school- based health education and/or as part of the science curriculum.
- Cardiovascular health education should be offered in places of religious worship and worksites where appropriate.
- Any CVD prevention programme should work closely with regional and local groups to promote policies likely to encourage healthier eating, reduce alcohol intake, reduce smoking and increase physical activity. These policies should also cover town planning, transport, food retailing and procurement.
- Organisations that might get involved in programme development could include statutory, public sector and civil

society groups such as charities, clubs, self-help and community groups such as Alcoholics Anonymous and Weight Watchers.

- Media campaigns can be useful but should be based on an acknowledged theoretical framework.

### 14.10.1 Responsibility for Population Based Approaches

**International level**: World Health Organisation (WHO), World Trade Organisation (WTO), European Union (EU). **National level**: Government departments, health authorities, health agencies, industries. **Regional level**: Authorities responsible for Traffic planning, Schools, construction of Public buildings. Responsibility must be shared between politicians, administrative authorities, health professionals and NGOs.

### 14.10.2 Recommendations for Action

**Food**

Changing dietary patterns from unhealthy to healthy foods and lowering daily total energy intake: **International level** WHO recommends salt intake less than 5g a day, saturated fat and sugar compromising less than 10% total energy (recently reduced to 5% total energy), elimination of trans fats. **National level** introducing taxes on unhealthy foods such as sugar, subsidising fruit and vegetables, restricting advertising of junk food (high in fat, salt and sugar), labelling to improve consumer information (traffic light schemes, healthy choice logos). **Regional level** Restrictions of availability (promoting nutritional criteria for schools, banning vending machines in schools, restricting fast food outlets near schools).

**Smoking**

Reducing smoking and second hand smoke exposure: **International level** WHO Framework Convention on Tobacco Control (FCTC) recommendations for smoke-free laws, already adopted by more than 170 countries, introduction of harmonisation of excise duties. **National level** Pricing and taxation (every 10% increase in retail price reduces consumption by 4%). Restrictions on sales to adolescents, possibly restrictions on sales to adults. Labelling with health warnings and plain packaging. Banning advertising, promotion and sponsorship. Media campaigns. Smoking bans in enclosed public places and workplaces. Banning designated smoking areas. Imposing penalties for breach of legislation. De-normalisation of smoking (by increasing public support for and compliance with smoking bans). **Regional level** Regulation of smoking in workplaces, educational centres and schools. Education in schools regarding harmful effects.

**Alcohol**

Reducing excessive alcohol consumption: **International level** WHO and EU recommend increased taxation, low legal limits for drivers, minimum purchase age and regulation of availability. **National level** Pricing and taxation (each 10% increase in retail price reduces consumption by between 4.6% and 8%), age limits for sales, drink-driving strategies, restricted sales outlets, reduced hours of sale, labelling with health warnings, restricting advertising, promotion and sponsorship. Reducing alcohol content of drinks. Introducing minimum pricing per unit. **Regional level** Regulation of consumption in workplaces, educational centres and schools. Education in schools regarding harmful effects.

## Physical Inactivity

Increased daily physical activity and decreased sedentary time. **International level** Change to environments that facilitates physical activity to fit into daily routine, publicise recommended guidelines for activities. **National and Regional** Taxing private motor transport, road user charges, higher parking fees and increasing availability of and subsidising public transport, introducing cycle and footpath lanes, narrowing roads in cities, creating increased places for physical activity, linking homes and schools by walking and cycling networks, encouraging use of stairs rather than lifts and escalators, designing school playgrounds to encourage varied physically active play, compulsory physical activity breaks in schools, encouraging employees to walk, cycle or use public transport to travel to and from work, introducing systematic breaks in sitting time.

**Reference:**

> Jorgensen Population-level changes to promote cardiovascular health Eur J Prev Card 2013; 20(3) 409-421

## 14.11 Additional Strategies

Nudging strategies, as used in advertising and space management in supermarkets, to gently push concepts so that the option obtained when the chooser does nothing is healthy rather than unhealthy.

Social support in stress prevention. Reducing social inequality in health.

**Reference:**

> ➢ Thaler Nudge. Improving decisions about health, wealth and happiness London: Penguin Books 2009

## 14.12 Legislative Measures

Legislative measures to reduce tobacco and alcohol usage, improve diet and increase physical activity are essential.

**Tobacco:**

Prohibiting sales to minors <18 years.

Prohibit tobacco advertising, promotion and sponsorship.

Banning smoking in enclosed public places.

Banning designated smoking areas.

Imposing penalties for breach of legislation.

Increasing tobacco tax.

Mandating non-branded plain cigarette packs and displaying health hazards on cigarette packs.

**Alcohol:**

Restricting sales to minors <18 years.

Restricted hours of permitted sale of alcohol.

Reducing alcohol content of drinks.

Increasing sales tax.

Introducing minimum pricing per unit.

Drunk driving laws - breathalysers.

Controlling advertising and sponsorships.

**Diet:**

Introducing sales tax on sugar-containing beverages and foods.

Limiting amount of saturated fat and trans fat in processed food.

Limiting salt content of processed food.

Standardising food labelling.

**Reference:**

➢ Prevention of Cardiovascular disease Nice public health
  guides 25

  http://www.nice.org.uk/guidance/ph25/resources/guidance-prevention-of-
  cardiovascular-disease-pdf

## 14.13 High Risk Approach

- The high risk approach however will depend mainly on
  health professionals in their direct work with individual
  patients.

- The high risk strategy seeks to identify the individuals who
  are at high risk because of marked elevation of either single
  or multiple risk factors. Targeted behavioral or
  pharmacological interventions will be needed in these cases.

- Risk assessment of individuals has been covered in detail in
  chapters 3 and 4.

- This approach provides the greatest risk reduction in
  individuals.

- Involvement of the family, spouse and children, will
  significantly improve the likely hood of effective lifestyle
  modification.

- In practice both population-based and high risk approaches
  should be introduced to achieve maximal results.

- Cost-effective and customized diagnostic and management algorithms should be developed for the treatment of all common CVD. These guidelines should be made widely available in the region.
- The availability of effective and affordable drugs, devices and procedures should be ensured.
- A teamwork approach is needed. Physicians will need support of nurses and allied health professionals such as dietitians, pharmacists, fitness trainers and smoking advisers.
- Referral chains should be established which should provide effective links between primary, secondary and tertiary health care centers whenever required.
- Greater emphasis must be placed on education and training in prevention for all health professionals at undergraduate and postgraduate levels. A 'train the trainers' approach should be adopted for promoting CVD prevention at the professional level.
- In order to provide a high risk approach alongside the population approach all physicians must commit the time to make a proper assessment and initiate preventive efforts. Physician's promotion of healthy habits including smoking cessation, reducing alcohol consumption, healthy eating, weight control, and increasing physical activity should be universal.

**References:**

➢ WHO Prevention of Cardiovascular Disease Guidelines for assessment and management of cardiovascular risk 2007 http://www.who.int/cardiovascular_diseases/guidelines/Full%20text.pdf

➢ Capewell S, Graham H (2010) Will Cardiovascular Disease Prevention Widen Health Inequalities? PLoS Med 7(8): e1000320. doi:10.1371/journal.pmed.1000320

## 14.14 The Essential Components of a CVD Control Programme

In practical terms the essential components of any CVD control programme are as shown below:

- Develop a health policy that will integrate population-based measures for CVD risk modification and cost-effective case management strategies for high risk groups.
- Ensure education and training for health professionals about prevention in general and risk factor management in particular.
- Introduce health education programmes for the general population including children, adults and families.
- Ensure efficient systems for assessing CVD risk factors in the population.
- Ensure efficient systems for monitoring CVD burden in the population.

**References:**

➢ Fuster V Promoting Cardiovascular Health in the Developing World: A Critical Challenge to Achieve Global Health Institute of Medicine (US) Committee on Preventing the Global

Epidemic of Cardiovascular Disease: Meeting the Challenges in Developing Countries National Academies Press (US); 2010
➢ NHS Health Check Programme Best Practice guidance 2013

## 14.14.1 CVD Programme Leadership

For any new programme to succeed there must be strong leadership and local ownership.

- Identify senior figures to act as champions.
- Identify and provide training for people to lead the CVD programme.
- Develop systems within local strategic partnerships and regional partnerships to agree shared priorities.
- It is therefore important at the outset to establish the above criteria and ensure they are applied.

## 14.14.2 Evaluating Impact

For prevention programmes to demonstrate success and ensure sustainability it is essential to monitor impact.

- Monitoring impact implies ensuring that evaluation is built in from the outset so that baseline measures can be made and outcomes monitored over time.
- Obtaining a fuller estimate of the burden of disease requires standardised morbidity data. Although gathering such data on a national basis would probably be impractical, obtaining prevalence data from valid cross-sectional sample surveys of selected communities and incidence data from selected

cohort studies would provide a reasonable basis for extrapolation.

- Health services of large organized sector industries may offer opportunities for convenient and cost-effective prospective studies and registries.
- Disease surveillance systems and CVD registries and data centres must be developed.
- In order for effective evaluation to take place it is also important that basic knowledge of epidemiology, biostatistics and public health should be core components of undergraduate and post-graduate education for all health professionals.

### 14.14.3 Implementing Change: Planning a Preventive Cardiology Programme

The aim of this chapter was to begin to consider how changes in professional behaviour and practice can be practically implemented in relevant healthcare settings.

You should now be able to:

- To confirm the need for establishing CVD prevention programme.
- To identify potential barriers to implementing necessary changes.
- To generate ideas to help overcome the barriers.
- To develop a plan towards local programme implementation.

- To consider methods to monitor and evaluate programme performance, for example disease registers and audits.

**References:**

➤ Services for Prevention of Cardiovascular disease NICE Commissioning guidelines CMG45 2012

➤ Saner H How to set up & run a cardiac rehabilitation programme EACPR 2012

### 14.15 How to reach high-risk Populations
### 14.15.1 Public Awareness Campaigns

To be effective they must periodically change their format, be frequently undertaken and be ongoing over many years.

Their aim is:

- To influence the general population to understand the social and economic problems caused by life-style factors, in particular alcohol, tobacco, unhealthy diet and insufficient exercise and to undertake measures to modify them and thus improve people's physical and psychological health and increase their earning capacity and life expectancy.
- To teach the public how to modify these factors.
- To demonstrate benefits of life-style modification.
- To encourage the public to attend their GP for cardiac and cancer risk assessment.
- In line with the objectives of UN and WHO the aim is to reduce incidence of and mortality from heart disease, stroke and cancers by 2% per annum.

## 14.15.2 Implementing Campaigns

i)   Involve wives and families.

ii)  Local media - introductory meeting with TV, radio, press.

iii) Involve VIPs and well-known individuals.

iv)  Community participation – meetings and demonstrations in shopping centres, factories, university, public administration buildings, army camps, schools, sports centres.

v)   Telephone hot-line.

vi)  Involvement of support groups such as AA and Weight Watchers.

vii) TV and radio programmes.

viii) Mobile phone texting.

ix)  Social media.

A Cochrane Review in 2011 which focused on counselling and educational interventions, and included 55 trials aimed at modifying one or more cardiovascular risk factors in the adult general population concluded that counselling and education to change behaviour do not reduce total or coronary heart disease mortality or clinical events in general populations. However, they noted that there were substantial shortcomings in the methods of the included trials, limiting the overall value of the findings.

Behavioural risk factor interventions are often labour-intensive and not sustainable over the long course, thus the effects tend to dwindle over time and require regular reinforcement.

**References:**

➢ Heneghan C. Considerable uncertainty remains in the evidence for primary prevention of cardiovascular disease [editorial]. Cochrane Database Syst Rev. 2011

➢ Tower Hamlets NHS Health checks 2014
www.healthcheck.nhs.uk/document.php?o=596

### 14.16 Managed Networks in General Practice

It has been demonstrated that linking several adjacent practices and employing common administrators and having common implementation of preventive programmes significantly increases patient uptake and improves achieved levels of results.

**Reference:**

➢ Robson Improving CVD using managed networks in general practice Br J Gen Pract 2014; 64:230-231

### 14.17 Other Useful Measures

• Opportunistic discussion with patients by GPs.

• Involving your patients in making healthcare decisions.

### 14.18 Nurse-led Programmes

Health Promotion workshops.

Multidisciplinary teams:

Core team: Nurse, Dietician, Physiotherapist, Cardiologist.

Supplementary team members: General practitioner, Psychologist, Social worker, Pharmacist, Occupational therapist, Diabetic specialist, Smoking-cessation specialist, Vocational counsellor, Sexual health specialist, Hospital Cardiologist and Specialist nurse.

**Reference:**

> Berra Nurse based models for CVD Prevention From research to clinical practice Jour Cardiovasc Nursing Aug 2011 Vol 26 No 4 546-555

## 14.19 Incentive Schemes

Debate continues whether or not incentive schemes, including financial rewards, have a significant role in motivating individuals to change their behaviour.

Certainly they played an effective part in North Karelia in Finland in the 1970s in reducing smoking and reducing consumption of dairy products. However, recent studies have found that the motivational effects wear off after a few months.

**References:**

> Puska P. Successful prevention of non-communicable diseases: 25 year experiences with North Karelia Project in Finland. Pub Health Med 2002; 4:5-7
> Jochelson Paying the patient, improving health using financial incentives Kings Fund 2007

## 14.20 Practical Implementation of Preventive Cardiology Programme

What do you actually do? You apply the basic clinical process of history taking, examination, investigation.

**History:**

Record age, gender, ethnicity, lifestyle history including smoking, alcohol, diet, exercise, stress, family history, past medical illness and medication.

**Physical examination:**

Check height, weight, waist circumference, pulse (rate and rhythm), blood pressure, urine dip stick test for protein and glucose, further examination of cardiovascular system, for example, assess heart size, heart sounds, carotid arteries, peripheral pulses, retinal fundi.

**Investigations:**

If necessary, on basis of history and examination, request blood tests for renal function, liver function, lipids, glucose, HbA1c.

**Risk assessment:**

Estimate the total risk of developing CVD over the following 10 years using QRISK2 or Heartscore.

**Advise patient** regarding life-style modification and prescribe appropriate prophylactic or therapeutic medication.

**Arrange** for regular monitoring and support.

### Questions and discussions

*Do effective CVD programmes already exist in the UK?*

*What are the barriers and how might they be overcome?*

*How can we engage local policy makers in a population approach?*

*How can we improve education and training in prevention for health professionals?*

*How can we improve risk factor detection and management in our practices and local clinics?*

*Who might lead our strategy?*

*How can we evaluate programmes?*

Consider the above questions and discuss them with colleagues.

## In Summary

- CVD prevention programmes have been established in the UK.
- Potential barriers to implementation must be identified and overcome.
- A population plus high risk approach is necessary.
- There must be attention to all levels of prevention that is primary, secondary and tertiary.
- Priority must be given to education, training and leadership.
- Methods must also be developed to monitor and evaluate programme performance.
- Obtaining a fuller estimate of the burden of disease requires standardised morbidity data.
- For effective evaluation to take place basic knowledge of epidemiology, biostatistics and public health should be core components of undergraduate and post-graduate education for all health professionals.
- Legislation to control tobacco and alcohol availability and usage, increase availability of healthy diets for adults and

children, and development of increased sports facilities must be introduced.

- Appropriate affordable medication must be available.

**This model is of universal application Worldwide.**

# Final Chapter

## 15. Case Discussions and Summary

Our final chapter focuses on case discussions relating to the content of the preceding chapters.

**Aim**

The aim of this chapter is to draw together learning from all previous chapters and consider practical implications.

**Objectives:**

- To reinforce the importance of identifying and treating cardiovascular risk factors in the community.
- To review the assessment of patients with cardiovascular risk.
- To review the management of patients with cardiovascular risk.
- To consider practical steps in order to establish local and national CVD prevention programmes.

**Topics**

1.  The Global problem of CVD

**Preventive Cardiology**

2.  CVD and Prevention
3.  CVD Risk Factors and Primary Prevention
4.  Clinical Risk Assessment for CVD

**Lifestyle Modification**

5.  Smoking

6. Alcohol
7. Diet and Weight
8. Physical activity
9. Stress

**Management of Medical Problems**

10. Hypertension
11. Cholesterol
12. Diabetes Mellitus

**Prevention Programmes**

13. Secondary and Tertiary Prevention
14. Preventive Cardiology Programme Planning and Implementing Change

**Summary**

15. Case discussions/Summary/Assessment

The above list reminds you of the areas covered in previous chapters.

## 15.1 Why is it important to Identify and Treat Cardiovascular Risk Factors?

In this chapter we review what has been previously covered and its practical application by discussing cases or situations which you have encountered in your own clinical practice.

We would like you to consider some prepared case vignettes and possibly discuss them for about 15 minutes with a colleague.

You can, of course, additionally or as an alternative, consider real cases you have come across in your professional career.

## Case 1

67 year old Asian female with diet-controlled Diabetes Mellitus. History of stroke. Family history of Ischaemic heart disease and stroke. Non-smoker. Medication Aspirin 75mgm daily. O/E Overweight, BP 146/72.

**What investigations would you do?**

**What is her overall CVD risk?**

**What should be done?**

## Case 2

55 year old man attends for repeat prescription. Hypertensive for 5 years, no secondary cause found. Irregularly attends doctor and BP control poor. Smoker. On Atenolol 100 mg daily, Captopril 25 mg tds, Bendroflumethazide 2.5 mg daily. BP 179/98. Heart rate 96 bpm. Urine dipstick ++ protein, Arterio-venous nipping on retinoscopy. ECG shows left ventricular hypertrophy. Creatinine is raised.

**Thoughts?**

## Case 3

58 year old woman with stable angina. Myocardial infarct 9 months ago. Ex-smoker. BP 142/86 mm Hg. Lipid profile: Total cholesterol 5.0 mmol/l, HDL 1.1 mmol/l, triglycerides 1.7 mmol/l. Current therapy: Aspirin 75 mg od, Ramipril 5 mg od, Atenolol 50 mg od, Simvastatin 40 mg nocte.

**Thoughts?**

## Case 4

76 year old male smoker has recovered well from a small stroke. 2 weeks later BP 180/100 mm Hg. Overweight, ex-smoker. O/E grade II retinopathy, 2 + blood and 2+ protein in urine.

**What would you do?**

Started on Perindopril + Indapamide. 1 week later: BP 137/85, 2+ blood and 2+ protein in urine, creatinine has risen from 120 to 197 mmol/l.

**Thoughts?**

## Case 5

30 year old woman with type 1 diabetes since childhood. Well controlled diabetes (HbA1c 6). Good lifestyle. BP 140/89. Lipid profile: Total cholesterol 5.5 mmol/l, HDL cholesterol 1.0, Triglycerides 1.6.

**Thoughts?**

## Case 6

86 year old active man. BP 174/92. Ex-smoker (stopped 10 years ago). Lipid profile: Total cholesterol 6.0 mmol/l, HDL cholesterol 1.1, Triglycerides 1.2.

**Thoughts?**

## Case 7

28 year old man. Overweight. BP 159/99 mm Hg. Ratio of Total:HDL cholesterol = 5.8. Smoker. Family history of premature CVD.

**Thoughts?**

## Case 8

68 year old woman. Stable claudication at 500 yards. BP 145/86. Ratio of Total:HDL cholesterol = 4.4. Ex-smoker.

**Thoughts?**

## Case 9

62 year old male baker with type 2 diabetes on Metformin. Smokes 15 cigarettes a day, overweight, drinks alcohol 56 units a week. BP 138/78 (3 months ago), 164/72 (1 month ago), 168/104 (2 weeks ago). Total cholesterol 6.3 mmol/l, HDL cholesterol 0.9 mmol/l, triglycerides 2.7 mmol/l. Fasting glucose 15 mmol/l.

**Thoughts?**

**Investigations?**

**Treatment?**

**Reference:**

> ➤ Case studies Dr Neil Chapman Centre for Circulatory Health Imperial College London

## In Summary

Over the course of this manual we hope that we have contributed to your understanding of CVD and agreed that:

- CVD is a major global healthcare problem in the UK and most developed and developing countries, resulting in serious human and economic costs.
- There is great potential for prevention at national, local and regional levels.
- To achieve this aim people must be shown how they can change their behaviour and modify their lifestyle.

- Making behavioural changes and modifying lifestyle is not easy, but is a very necessary exercise.
- Health promotion and disease prevention should receive greater emphasis in the training of all health professionals.
- The general population should be regularly reminded by health professionals about risk factors and healthy lifestyle.
- Widespread and repeated educational programmes for adults and children should be introduced in schools and workplaces.
- Organised and regularly monitored programmes are needed to identify individuals at risk.
- Risk assessment should be undertaken on a holistic basis.
- Greater priority should be given to risk factor management.

### Finale - a salutary thought

A woman walks up to an old man sitting in a chair on his porch. "*I couldn't help but notice how happy you look*", she said. "*What's your secret for a long, happy life?*"

"*I smoke three packs a day, drink a case of beer, eat fatty foods, and never, ever exercise*", he replied. "*Wow, that's amazing*", she said, "*How old are you?*"

"*Twenty-six.*"

# 16. Synopsis
# Preventive Cardiology

More people in the world die each year from CVD than from any other cause. The developing countries contribute a greater share to the global burden of CVD than the developed countries.

Most deaths are avoidable by targeting risk factors such as smoking, alcohol, obesity, physical inactivity, hypertension, diabetes, raised lipids and stress.

There are two complimentary approaches to preventing CVD. The Population approach aimed at changing society's behaviour largely by legislative measures. The High Risk approach aimed at modifying individuals' lifestyle.

We must aim to reduce morbidity and mortality from CVD by 2% per annum.

This manual has demonstrated how you can set up preventive cardiology programmes in general practices.

The ultimate aim is to assist the public to modify their behaviour and lifestyles.

Many questions remain unanswered, probably most importantly:
*How can we most accurately assess cardiac risk?*
*How can we best influence individuals to modify their lifestyle?*

## Appendix A
## 17. Preventive Cardiology in Russia

Let us now look at the effect of CVD in a European middle income developed country (Appendix D). Recently revised to upper income.

CVD is the main cause of death in people under the age of 70 years and is responsible for 35% of all male and female deaths in Russia.

### 17.1 Demographic Data for Russia

- In 2010 the population of the Russian Federation was 142,958,164. Until 2010 this population was decreasing, due to a reduced birth rate, imbalance between immigration and emigration and a continuing high male mortality rate.

- Non-communicable diseases in Russia account for 82% of all deaths, and 62% of these deaths are caused by CVD. CVD is responsible for 51% of all deaths in the Russian Federation, approximately 600,000 male deaths annually, and for one third of all deaths in the 25-64 age group. Largely due to these CVD-related deaths until 2010 the Russian population was falling annually by 0.5%.

- In 2010 death rate from CVD in Russia was 915 men and 517 women per 100,000 population.

- Although WHO has not published any data relating to the Russian Federation more recent than 2011, there have been some newer more promising figures emerging from the Russian Federation. Latest Russian Federation Health Ministry figures show that, over the course of the four years

2010 to 2014, life expectancy has improved for males from 60.5 years to 63.3 years, and for females from 73.3 years to 75 years.

- Overall mortality rates were down by 5.9% from 15.2 per 1,000 in 2006 to 14.3 per 1,000 in 2010, with a further fall to 13 per 1,000 in 2013. More specifically, mortality rates for circulatory disease have reduced by 7%. Incidence of Strokes has reduced by 20% and overall CVD by 5%.

- This demonstrates that these rates can be significantly reduced by introduction of a few straight-forward but very effective measures such as public awareness campaigns, health education, Health Centres for screening for CVD, and also by the development of local and regional vascular centres, aimed at treating people with acute myocardial infarctions and stroke, as rapidly as possible.

**References:**

- Dying too Young World Bank 1-15 2005
- Kim AS Global Variation in the Relative Burden of Stroke and IHD Circulation. 2011 Jul 19; 124(3):314-23
- Ministry of Health Russian Federation Rosstat 2013-2015

### 17.2 The Burden of CVD in Russia

- In most European countries life expectancy is increasing, however the life expectancy in countries such as Russia and Ukraine actually dropped in the 50 years 1960 to 2010.

- From 1945 to 1960 mortality improved considerably in Eastern Europe because of improvements in housing and hygiene, and the control of communicable diseases. At that time there was only a small discrepancy between life expectancy in Eastern and Western countries of Europe.

- By the 1970s and 1980s life expectancy in Western Europe started to significantly improve because of work and lifestyle modification and reduction in deaths from NCD, but this was not so in Eastern Europe, leading to a wider gap between the two regions.

- After the fall of the Soviet Union in 1991 there was a sharp decline in life expectancy in the Russian Federation and other Eastern European countries, especially amongst men. Following a small improvement in the late 1990s there was a decline again with a leveling off in the mid-2000s. The gap between these Eastern and Western European countries continued to grow.

- Much of the reduction in life expectancy came about because of lifestyle factors, such as poor diet, inadequate exercise, excessive smoking, high alcohol consumption and increased levels of stress leading to increased CVD and other smoking and alcohol-related diseases, as well as accidents and injuries.

- Until 2010 the Russian population of approximately 143 million was decreasing annually by 700,000. CVD accounts for some 600,000 male deaths each year in Russia. If this rate were to continue there could be a fall in Russia's population by as much as 23% by 2050, clearly with potentially disastrous socio-economic consequences.

Measures were introduced in 2012 to reduce the fall in population.

- In 2006 life expectancy at birth for men in the Russian Federation was just over 60 years, compared to Chinese men who had a life expectancy at birth of 72.2 years. Russian women at birth could expect to live to an average age of 73.3, compared to 75.8 for women in China. The rates in India were similar to those in the Russian Federation, but in India lives were cut short more often for different reasons. As well as having high rates of non-communicable diseases, poor living standards, poor housing and poor hygiene conditions mean that in India there is a higher prevalence of communicable diseases, which additionally accounts for more deaths. Male life expectancy in Russia has now increased to 63.3 years.

- The death rate from CVD and Diabetes in the Russian Federation and the whole of the Eastern European block remains high, in comparison with Western Europe and North America and even much of Asia.

- Recent reports show in 2014 an increase in overall life expectancy to 70.8 years and fall in CVD mortality to 653 per 100,000 population (49.9% of total deaths).

- CVD mortality rates declined by 30% between 2003 (927/100,000) and 2014 (653/100,000).

**References:**

➤ Nichols M et al Cardiovascular disease in Europe 2014: epidemiological update European Heart Journal doi:10.1093/eurheartj/ehu299

➤ Rosstat 2013-15

## 17.3 The Impact of CVD in Russia

- CVD is the major cause of premature death in Russia. It is an important cause of disability and contributes substantially to the escalating costs of health care.

- The falling population has already caused serious problems at personal and family level by increasing stress, depression and alcoholism, creating more widows and thus destabilising families and reducing family income.

- At the national level CVD causes increased medical costs, reduced productivity and tax revenue, decreased savings, increased absenteeism from work, fewer workers, potential regional disparities, fewer military conscripts and increased risks of potential instability.

**Reference:**

➤ Dying Too Young, World Bank 15-16 2005

## 17.4 Tobacco Smoking in Russia

While prevalence of smoking has been declining in England and the rest of the world, until recently prevalence in Russia had increased. This increase was due to the massive increase in women smokers in the decade from 12.6% in 1999/2000 to 21.7% in 2009.

Compared to the rest of world there is currently a tobacco pandemic in Russia. Russia has one of the highest rates of tobacco consumption in the world. In 2009 a total of 39.1% of the population in Russia smoked; 63% of men and 30% of women were smokers. Recent 2015 figures show a reduction by 17% of total smokers and a fall in percentage of male smokers to 60%.

Compare this with smokers forming 21% of the population in England.

**References:**

  ➤ European health for all database, WHO Regional Office for Europe. http://data.euro.who.int/hfabd 2012
  ➤ Ministry of Health and Social Development of the Russian Federation and Federal State Statistics Service (RosStat). The Global Adult Tobacco Survey (GATS) Russian Federation 2009 Country Report
  ➤ Rosstat 2013-15

- Tobacco use is the third leading cause of premature death in Russia and the average life expectancy in Russian males is more than 10 years less than for Western European males.
- Smoking accounts for 92% of all deaths due to lung cancer, and for 27% of all deaths due to CVD. 330,000-400,000 Russians die each year from smoking related illnesses. Male smoking attributed deaths in 2009: All causes 22%, Lung cancer 92%, COPD 73%, Vascular 27%.
- In spite of the high prevalence of smoking Russians appear to be knowledgeable about the risks. 90% believe that smoking causes

serious illness, and high percentages are aware of the main diseases caused by smoking. 60% say they are interested in quitting, but only 32% made an attempt to quit in the last year and only 32% were advised to quit by a health professional.

**References:**

➤ Gerasimenko N, Zaridze D, Sakharova G, eds. Health and Tobacco: Facts and Figures. 2007

➤ Federal State Statistics Service. Life expectancy at birth. Moscow, Russia, 2008

➤ Peto R, Lopez A, et al. Mortality from smoking in developed countries 1950 – 2009. http://www.ctsu.ox.ac.uk/~tobacco/

➤ GATS Russian Federation 2009. MPOWER Summary Indicators

➤ European health for all database, WHO Regional Office for Europe 2014. http://data.euro.who.int/hfabd

➤ Ministry of Health and Social Development of the Russian Federation and Federal State Statistics Service (RosStat). The Global Adult Tobacco Survey (GATS) Russian Federation 2009 Country Report.

### 17.4.1 Tobacco Control in Russia

- The WHO Framework Convention on Tobacco Control (WHO FCTC) was adopted in 2003 and signed by 168 States. It was ratified in 2008 by the Russian Federation.

- Russia in June 2013 introduced measures to restrict smoking in workplaces, on aircraft, trains and municipal transport as well as in schools, hospitals, cultural institutions and government buildings, requiring specially designated smoking areas to be set up and restaurants and cafes to set up no-smoking areas.

- It is proposed to prohibit tobacco advertising and promotion, increase cigarette prices from 17 to 61 roubles per pack and introduce minimum prices and empower regional governments with tobacco control powers.

- Treatment programmes and facilities would also benefit from up-dating, but there is a toll free telephone quit line and smoking cessation support available in some health clinics and primary care facilities.

**Reference:**

➢ Tobacco control in Russian Federation COP6 Ministry of Healthcare Russian Federation 2014

### 17.5 Alcohol in Russia

- A recent WHO report stated that Russians were the 4th heaviest drinkers of alcohol in the world after Moldova, the Czech Republic and Hungary. 20% of male deaths and 6% of female deaths in the Russian Federation are linked to alcohol.

- Alcohol consumption in Russia is almost double the critical level set by the WHO.

- In Russia average alcohol consumption was reported at 18 litres of 40% spirit per person per year in 2009.

- Alcoholic cardiomyopathy constitutes half of all female and a quarter of male CVD deaths classified as alcoholic in age group 30-49 years in Russia.

- Drinking cheap surrogate alcohol products such as perfume, detergents or industrial cleaning products and binge drinking (zapoy) are common problems in Russia.
- Following introduction of new laws and restrictions, there has been a measurable reduction in alcohol sales.

**References:**

➤ D Leon et al Hazardous alcohol drinking and premature mortality in Russia: a population based case-control study The Lancet, Volume 369, Issue 9578, Pages 2001 - 2009, 16 June 2007

➤ Sidorenkov et al Premature CV Mortality and alcohol consumption before death in Archangelsk Russia Int Jr Epidem 10.1093/ije/dyr 145 2010

### 17.5.1 Alcohol Licensing Laws in Russia

Some recent changes in Russian laws should have an impact on high rates of alcohol consumption. These include: Restriction of drinking in some public places such as parks, gardens, stairways and elevators. The reclassifying of beer from a soft drink to an alcoholic drink in January 2013. Restriction of times of sale (for example in Moscow alcohol cannot be sold between 10pm and 10am). Restriction on places of sale. Licensing laws for imported alcohol. Age restrictions. Increased excise duty on the sale of alcohol and price regulation.

When fully implemented these measures should significantly reduce alcohol consumption in Russia.

**Reference:**

➢ Loginov M New Russian laws: no chance of a drink or smoke Open Democracy March 2013

https://www.opendemocracy.net/...russia/.../new-russian-laws

## 17.6 Diet and Obesity in Russia

- Amongst Russian adults aged 25-64 years 48% of males and 52% of females are overweight (BMI >25).

- Between 2008 and 2010 the percentage of obese Muscovites increased from 17.3% to 38.2%. It is predicted that by 2020 31% males and 26% females will be obese.

- The Organisation for Economic Cooperation & Development released figures in 2009, which showed that just under half of adults in the Russian Federation have weights which are classified as obese.

- As in the UK increasing rates of obesity, at all ages, associated with high fat/low fibre diet, alongside with a high alcohol intake in Russia, are an important risk factor in maintaining high levels of CVD.

- There is wide regional variation in diet and alcohol consumption in different regions in Russia.

- A CINDI (Countrywide Integrated Non-communicable Disease Intervention) programme survey of eating and drinking habits, using a random population sample of 25-64 year olds, was carried out in the Ural region of Russia between 2003 and 2005. This showed that the eating and drinking habits of the people in that region were not as healthy as they could be. Figures suggest that the high fat/low fibre diet, alongside a high alcohol intake, could well be contributing to the high rates of CVD in the region.

**References:**

- ➢ CINDI (Countrywide Integrated Non-communicable Disease Intervention) programme survey, which was carried out using a random population sample of 25-64 year olds, between 2003 and 2005
- ➢ RIA Novosti interview Leonid Lobaznik Chief physician Moscow Healthcare department 2010
- ➢ OECD Third Lancet series on Chronic Diseases - Russian Federation 2010
- ➢ WHO Global Health Observatory Data Repository Nutrition, Physical Activity & Obesity in the Russian Federation 2013

## 17.7 Physical Activity in Russia

Survey studies have shown that in general Russian men, women and children, do not engage in enough physical activity in their weekly routines. A survey conducted in Russian cities in 2001-2002 showed that only 6% of Russians regularly participate in sport fitness programmes. 81% of men and 86% of women aged 25-64 years had low physical activity during their free time.

Russian boys and girls spend 28 hours a week on sedentary activities. 70% Russian youth meet guideline 1 requirements for physical activity and <45% for guidelines 2.

**References:**

- ➢ Potemkina RA, Glazunov IS, Kuznetsova OYu, Petrukhin IS, Frolova YeV, Kudina YeA, et al. Examination of the spread of behavioral risk factors among the population of Moscow, Saint Petersburg, and Tver by telephone questioning. Profilac Zabol Ukrep Zdor 2005; 3:3-15

➤ Petrukhin IS, Lunina EY. Cardiovascular disease risk factors and mortality in Russia: challenges and barriers. Public Health Reviews. 2011; 33: Epub

➤ Levin et al Patterns of physical activity among Russian youth Russian Longitudinal Monitoring Survey European Journal of Public Health 09/1999; 9(3).1999

➤ Goskomstat Russian State Statistics Committee 2002

➤ CINDI Behavioural Risk Factor Surveillance System Development in Russia in 2004

The Russian Federation are yet to bring out their own specific guidelines, but an action plan for physical education was included in school curricula in 2009.

## 17.8 Stress in Russia

According to the Interheart study, adverse psycho-social conditions are arguably associated with an increased risk of myocardial infarct and contribute to 35% of population attributable risk in Russia.

**References:**

➤ Interheart study Rosengren Lancet 2004; 364:953-962

➤ Pajak CVD in Central & Eastern Europe Public Health Reviews Vol 33 No 2 416-435 2012

## 17.9 Hypertension in Russia

• 12 million Russians have high blood pressure.

- The prevalence of hypertension in Russia is 85.4 per 1000 population, of which Essential hypertension prevalence is 75.7 per 1000 and Secondary 9.6 per 1000.
- There is considerable regional and ethnic variation. For example in Ufa in the South West Ural mountains the prevalence is 109.7 per 1000 population.

**Reference:**

- ➢ Petrukhin IS, Lunina EY. Cardiovascular disease risk factors and mortality in Russia: challenges and barriers. Public Health Reviews. 2012; 33:436-49

### 17.10 Drug Treatment of Hypertension in Russia

The Russian national guidelines for hypertension are based on ESC (European Cardiology Society) and ESH (European Society of Hypertension) guidelines 2007.

Hypertension is categorised as High normal/Grade1/Grade2/Grade3

**Reference:**

- ➢ Karpov New guidelines for hypertension in Russia--a priority of combined treatment Ter Arkh. 2012; 84(1):61-4. [Article in Russian]

### 17.11 Cholesterol in Russia

In 2008 in Russia 54 million people had raised total cholesterol levels (total population 143 million). The proportion of the population with raised cholesterol levels remains high.

During the period 1989-1997 cholesterol levels in Russia were among the lowest in Europe.

**Reference:**

➤ WHO Monica project Geographical variations in major risk factors of CHD WHO Stat Q 41: 115 -40 2003

## 17.12 Diabetes in Russia

Russia has the fifth largest number of diabetics in the world. 6% of the population, 8 million people, are thought to have diabetes. 90% of these have Type 2 diabetes. The prevalence of Type 2 diabetes in Russia is 87.8 per 1000 population. Possibly 50% of cases are undiagnosed. Several risk factors are highly prevalent in those people not reporting a diagnosis of diabetes.

**References:**

➤ Diabetes in Russia. Problems & Solutions 2008
➤ Russia National & Wellness Survey 2011

### Summary

- The causes of CVD and associated risk factors in Russia largely mirror those of the rest of the World.
- In large part Russia's falling population is due to early male deaths from CVD.
- Levels of tobacco smoking and alcohol consumption are amongst the highest in the developed world.
- Many people in the Russian Federation eat unhealthy diets and take little exercise.

- The incidence of hypertension and diabetes, diagnosed and undiagnosed are high.
- However steps have been introduced to counter many of these risk factors and have already shown significant improvements in morbidity, mortality and life expectancy.

# Appendix B
# 18. Basic Cardiology
## Key Points

In case we have forgotten let us briefly remind ourselves of basic cardiac anatomy and physiology.

## 18.1 What are Cardiovascular Diseases?

CVD covers all the diseases of the heart and circulation including coronary heart disease (CHD) (angina and heart attack), stroke and transient ischaemic attacks (TIA).

CVD are diseases of the heart and blood vessels that are caused by atheroma. Patches of atheroma are small fatty deposits which develop within the intima of arteries. A patch of atheroma (plaque) narrows the lumen of the artery and reduces the blood flow through the artery. Sometimes plaques may rupture stimulating blood clots to form over the atheroma causing further obstruction which may critically affect the blood supply distally. Depending on the site of the atheromatous plaque the clinical presentation may manifest as heart attack, angina, stroke or peripheral vascular disease.

**Reference:**
> WHO Cardiovascular diseases (CVDs) Fact sheet No. 317 Updated January 2015

## 18.2 The Anatomy of the Heart

- The heart is a pump made of muscle. It has four chambers (right atrium and ventricle, left atrium and ventricle). The right side receives deoxygenated blood from the vena cava and pumps it to the lungs (Pulmonary circulation). The left side receives oxygenated blood from the lungs and pumps it to the rest of the body (Systemic circulation).

- The heart muscle, the myocardium, is made up of specific muscle cells, which have electrical connections. This means that when each muscle cell contracts, it leads to a wave of depolarisation across the whole myocardium.

**Reference:**

> Texas Heart Institute Normal heart anatomy
> www.nlm.nih.gov/medlineplus/ency/imagepages/8672.htm

### 18.3 The Cardiac Cycle

- The cardiac cycle consists of two stages: systole and diastole.
- The cycle starts when the pace-maker cells in the sino-atrial node, situated in the right atrium, rhythmically depolarise across the atria, causing the atria to contract. The depolarisation arrives at the atrio-ventricular node. The atrio-ventricular node then causes rhythmical depolarisation down the Bundle of His, which branches from the base of the ventricles and spreads across the myocardium.
- The ventricles contract from the bottom upwards, forcing blood through the valves into the pulmonary and aorta arteries – this is the phase of Systole.
- The phase of Diastole occurs when the myocardium is resting, and the atria fill with blood – either from the vena cava or the pulmonary artery.

**Reference:**

➤ Cardiovascular physiology concepts Cardiac cycle

   http://www.cvphysiology.com/Heart%20Disease/HD002.htm

## 18.4 The Coronary Circulation

*Corona* is a Latin word meaning crown, and it aptly describes the vasculature supplying the cardiac tissues.

- The name of each artery or branch is determined by the distal territory supplied by the artery, rather than its origin.

- The right coronary artery (RCA) runs along the atrio-ventricular groove, and supplies much of the right ventricular wall.

- In 90% of patients, the RCA supplies the posterior descending coronary artery branch, which supplies the crux of the heart (the junction of the walls of the four chambers).

- The Right Coronary Artery forms branches which supply much of the atria, as well as the sinus node.

- The Left Coronary Artery (LCA) divides into the Left Anterior Descending (LAD), and the Circumflex arteries.

- The LAD runs in the interventricular groove splitting into anterior septal perforating branches. It also supplies the antero-lateral wall of the left ventricle. The Circumflex artery runs along the atrioventricular groove and then posteriorly to the posterior aspect of the crux of the heart.

- Although anastomoses form, significant obstruction of a major branch will lead to ischaemic damage of the part of the muscle that branch supplied. The cardiac muscle has very limited capacity for anaerobic metabolism, so is at particular risk of ischaemic damage.

**Reference:**

➢ Coronary Anatomy & Blood Flow

  http://www.cvphysiology.com/Blood%20Flow/BF001.htm

## Appendix C

## 19. Pathophysiology of Ischaemic Heart Disease

In order to explore what pathology can occur within the cardiovascular system and put the condition in a scientific context, we will spend some time reminding you of the biomedical theory behind CVD.

Then we shall consider which organs CVD damages, and the consequences of this damage.

### 19.1 Atherosclerosis

This can occur throughout the vascular tree including: Coronary arteries, around the heart valves, in the aorta, Cerebral blood vessels, Peripheral blood vessels. It begins early in life and progresses steadily.

Atherosclerosis (atheroma) is a disease process of the large and medium-sized muscular arteries. There are several features in the development of atherosclerosis including endothelial dysfunction, vascular inflammation, and the build-up of materials such as lipids, cholesterol and calcium deposits in the intima of the vessel wall. This build up leads to plaque formation and vascular remodelling, which in turn results in luminal obstruction, abnormalities of blood flow and eventually reduced oxygen delivery to end organs.

**Reference:**

> Peter Libby et al Progress and challenges in translating the biology of atherosclerosis Nature 473,317–325 Fig 1 2011

### 19.1.1 Development of Arteriosclerosis

- The mechanism of atherogenesis remains incompletely understood. There appears to be a multi-factorial and complex interaction between a number of pathophysiological processes, including vasomotor function, the thrombogenicity of the blood vessel wall, cellular inflammation, the coagulation cascade and fibrinolytic system.

- At this point in time, the most widely-accepted theory is known as the 'response to injury' theory. The response to injury theory proposes that endothelial injury causes vascular inflammation and a fibro-proliferative response. Likely causative agents of endothelial injury include low-density lipoproteins, cholesterol, toxins including those produced by smoking, infection, hyperglycaemia, and hyper homocystinaemia.

- Once this process has happened, circulating leukocytes permeate the intima of the vessel wall, and these macrophages act as scavenger cells, taking up LDL cholesterol and forming the typical foam cell of early atherosclerosis.

- As lipid accumulation progresses, and with the additional proliferation of smooth muscle cells, the fatty streak can become a fibrous plaque. Following that a fibrous cap develops overlying the foam cells, extracellular lipid cells and necrotic core. Progression of the plaque leads to luminal narrowing and blood flow abnormalities. Impairment of blood flow occurs once the luminal narrowing becomes greater than 50-70% of the lumen diameter. In the event of increased metabolic and oxygen demands by the end organ, the flow impairment will result in symptoms of inadequate blood supply and oxygenation.

- Plaque rupture occurs because of weakening of the fibrous cap. A plaque rupture can result in thrombus formation (which in turn can lead to emboli). Alternatively, the rupture can lead to partial or complete occlusion of the blood vessel in which it is sited.

- The lesions of atherosclerosis do not site themselves in a totally random fashion. Atherosclerotic plaques tend to form in regions of branching and curvature of the vessels. These locations tend to denote places of irregular geometry, as well as areas where the blood flow experiences a significant change in velocity or direction of flow. It is thought that the turbulence this produces, in addition to the decreased sheer stress, results in atherogenesis in the coronary arteries, important sites of the thoracic and abdominal aorta, and large conduit vessels of the legs.

**Reference:**

➤ Peter Libby et al Progress and challenges in translating the biology of atherosclerosis Nature 473,317–325 Fig 2 2011

### 19.1.2 Length of time for Atheroma to form

| | | | |
|---|---|---|---|
| Stage 1 | Age | 0 | No atheroma |
| Stage 2 | Age | 10-20 | Fatty streaks in intima |
| Stage 3 | Age | 20-30 | Formation fibrous plaques |
| Stage 4 | Age | 30-40 | Calcification, haemorrhage, ulceration, thrombosis formation |
| Stages 5 & 6 | Age | 40-70 | Infarct, Stroke, Gangrene, Aneurysm |

- There are 6 stages or types of atherosclerotic lesions which usually take at least 40 years to develop.
- The first two stages occur in the $1^{st}$ to $2^{nd}$ decade, the second two stages develop from the $3^{rd}$ decade, and the last two stages from the $4^{th}$ decade onwards.
- The first fatty streaks can be found in the aorta shortly after birth, and appear in an increasing number in individuals between the ages of 8-18.
- More advanced or extensive lesions develop once someone reaches the age of 25, and the lesions progress in extent and complexity with advancing years. Organ specific manifestations increase with age well into the $5^{th}$ and $6^{th}$ decade.
- The first four stages relate very closely to lipid accumulation and deposit and up to stage three atherosclerotic formations can be silent.
- The final three stages may continue to be clinically silent, but can become overt at any stage or point in time.

- Reversal can be achieved, we have discussed how this can be done throughout the manual.

**Reference:**

➢ AHA Conference Atherosclerosis Vascular disease Pathophysiology Circulation 2004; 109: 2617-2625

### 19.1.3 Interplay between Risk Factors and Pathogenesis

Atherosclerosis (Atheroma) is at the centre of a complex web and network of metabolic and circulatory conditions.

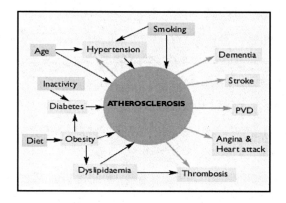

The risk factors - age, smoking, inactivity, diet and obesity, dyslipidaemia, alcohol and clinical disease - hypertension, diabetes all play a part in the development of atheroma. Atheroma has a significant role in development of angina and heart attack, stroke, peripheral vascular disease, thrombosis and dementia. There is an on-going inter-play between risk factors and pathogenesis.

During the course of this manual you will have learned in detail about the different risk factors for developing atherosclerosis and

CVD. Some conditions such as hypertension act both as causes and consequences of atheroma.

**Reference:**

> Boudi B et al Risk Factors for Coronary Artery Disease emedicine.medscape.com/article/164163 2014

## 19.2 Hypertension

- Hypertension is diagnosed when a person has a BP of >140/90 on at least 3 occasions, recorded 4 weeks each apart.

- Hypertension is generally a condition without symptoms, which makes it difficult to explain to the patient that it is something worthy of attention or treatment. However, we know that hypertension creates huge risks and serious implications for cardiovascular health.

- The risk associated with rising blood pressure is continuous, with each 2mm Hg increase of systolic blood pressure associated with a 7% increased risk of mortality from ischaemic heart disease and a 10% increased risk of stroke. This increased risk is brought about by the higher haemodynamic load, increased vascular resistance, and atherogenesis causing end-organ damage to vital organs such as the heart, brain or kidneys.

- Hypertension may be primary – in other words a result of genetic components and environmental components – or secondary as a result of particular conditions, for example renal disease, vasculitis, endocrine conditions, or specific drugs.

- In general, 50% of the world's population over the age of 60 are thought to have hypertension, which means that overall an estimated 20% of the world's total adult population are affected.

- Whether or not end-organ damage results from hypertension depends of course on the extent (and response to treatment) of the hypertension, but we also know that there are certain factors which are independent of the blood pressure control – such as obesity, salt intake, genetic make-up – which means that some patients with well-controlled hypertension will develop end-organ damage and some patient with the same control of hypertension, will not.

- Because of the complex inter-relationship between all these predisposing factors, it is difficult to predict how long uncontrolled hypertension will take to damage end organs, but generally speaking the timeframe is years rather than months.

**Reference:**

➢ Schmieder R End Organ Damage In Hypertension Dtsch Arztebl Int. 2010 December; 107(49): 866–873

### 19.3 End - Organ Damage
### 19.3.1 The Heart
### 19.3.2 Coronary/Ischaemic Heart Disease

Atherosclerosis causes plaque formation, luminal occlusion, vascular remodelling, and abnormal blood flow, resulting in Acute

Coronary Syndrome (ACS), or Acute Myocardial Infarction (AMI). Approximately one third of people who experience an AMI in the US will not survive it.

The survivors of an AMI have a poor prognosis. They carry between 1.5 to 15-fold increase in likelihood of mortality and morbidity compared to the normal population. Up to 25% of men and 38% of women in the US die in the year following an AMI. Additionally, 7% of men and 6% of women die suddenly, 22% of men and 46% of women are disabled with chronic heart failure, and 8% of men and 11% of women go on to have a stroke. The prognosis of patients with atherosclerosis is dependent on a number of variables, including the presence of ischaemia, arrhythmias, impaired left ventricular function, the aggressiveness of risk reduction and compliance with medication.

### 19.3.3 Heart Failure

Heart Failure can result from ischaemic damage to the heart which leads to reduced myocardial function, but there are many other causes too. These include amongst others hypertension, arrhythmias, thyroid disease, alcohol, cardiomyopathy and valvular disease.

Cardiac failure can be categorised into left ventricular impairment, or diastolic dysfunction – which in the past was termed right sided heart failure, and which may be more difficult to identify (as changes may be absent on echocardiography). Diagnosis is made by a combination of symptoms, signs and the gold standard investigation is an echocardiagram. There is now a blood test available called pro-Beta Naturetic Peptide which has a high specificity, and if negative, almost certainly rules out the likelihood of heart failure. There are several pharmacological interventions available which have been shown to improve rates of mortality for patients who have heart failure.

**References:**

- ➢ Burke AP Pathophysiology of acute myocardial infarct Med Clin North Am. 2007 Jul; 91(4):553-72; ix
- ➢ Kemp CD The pathophysiology of heart failure Cardiovasc Pathol. 2012 Sep-Oct; 21(5):365-71

### 19.3.4 The Brain

### 19.3.5 Cerebrovascular Accidents or Strokes

Strokes (CVA) are responsible for 33% of deaths annually worldwide, and they are the third leading cause of death in many western countries.

The equivalent of CVD in the brain is known as cerebrovascular disease. The pathological processes are the same, namely atherosclerosis and hypertension, and these can lead to ischaemic, or haemorrhagic sequelae. Hypertension is the biggest risk factor for stroke, but the other CVD risk factors, discussed in the manual, also play a major role in causing strokes.

A cerebrovascular accident (stroke) is characterised by a sudden loss of blood supply to a part of the brain tissue, resulting in a corresponding loss of neurological function. This loss of blood supply can be caused by thrombosis, emboli, or haemorrhage. The former two are much more common than the latter – 80% are ischaemic compared with 20% being haemorrhagic.

The Trial of Org 10172 in Acute Stroke Treatment (TOAST) divided ischaemic stroke into 3 main categories:

- Large artery infarction, thrombotic in nature and caused by in situ atherosclerosis in the carotid, vertebro-basilar, or cerebral arteries.
- Small vessel infarcts, known as lacunar.
- Cardio-embolic – where an embolus from the heart is carried into the cerebral vasculature and causes a stroke. This is the common causes of recurrent strokes and accounts for 20% of acute strokes. Risk factors for these strokes include Atrial Fibrillation and recent cardiac surgery. They also carry a particularly poor prognosis.

Whilst it has been established that hypertension is the greatest risk factor for Cerebro-vascular accidents, the mechanisms which link the two are complex and multi-faceted. A high intra-luminal pressure can cause alteration and damage of the endothelium and smooth muscle in the cerebral arteries. This can in turn lead to thrombotic and ischaemic lesions forming, it can result in localised oedema, or predispose to intra-cerebral haemorrhages. Moreover, as already discussed, it can accelerate atherosclerosis formation both inside the brain increasing the risk of developing stenoses and occlusions, but also in extra-cranial arteries, potentially resulting in emboli formation which then occlude intra-cranial vessels.

### 19.3.6 Transient Ischaemic Attack (TIA)

A TIA or 'mini stroke' is caused by a temporary disruption in the blood supply to part of the brain. However, unlike a stroke, the effects of a TIA only last for a few minutes and are usually fully resolved within 24 hours.

**Reference:**

➢ Giraldo E Ischemic Stroke Merck Manual 2015

### 19.3.7 Vascular Dementia

Vascular dementia is the second most common form of dementia after Alzheimer's Disease.

Again, there are a variety of sub-types and causes – from multiple brain infarcts, to one single strategic infarct (affecting a significant area of the brain), to vascular dementia from lacunar or haemorrhagic lesions. Silent damage can also be caused by hypertension and atherosclerosis leading to small vessel disease.

Brain damage to the white cerebral hemispheres, and deep grey nuclei are associated with the cognitive decline. Often people will have a mix of vascular and Alzheimer's dementia. Clinically, cognitive impairment will progress slowly over time. When associated with multi-infarcts the deterioration is typically step-wise.

**Reference:**

➢ Alagiakrishnan K Vascular Dementia Pathophysiology Medscape 2015

### 19.3.8 The Kidneys

Chronic kidney disease (CKD) is a growing health problem worldwide associated with high costs and a poor outcome. It causes increased deaths from CVD – people with CKD are 16 to 40 times more likely to die from CVD, than to progress to kidney failure.

Often chronic kidney disease is clinically silent, and so vigilance on the part of the clinician is essential in picking up patients who may be at risk. If not diagnosed early the prognosis for chronic kidney disease is poorer, and renal replacement therapy (for example, dialysis) is expensive and once patients have reached that stage their morbidity and mortality substantially increases.

Hypertensive nephropathy can result in chronic renal failure and it is the major cause of chronic kidney disease worldwide. It is often clinically silent and generally occurs after approximately 15-20 years of hypertension.

One theory states that increased glomerular pressure leads to glomerular capillary damage which can eventually lead to widespread glomerulosclerosis. Once again, the same risk factors which cause other system vascular disease are implicated with renal disease – namely – hypertension, smoking, hyperlipidaemia, diabetes. Of course there are many other causes of chronic kidney disease but we are not going to focus on those.

Early damage can be detected using Estimated Glomerular Filtration Rate (eGFR) as a blood test and urinary Albumin/Creatinine Ratio as a measure of microalbuminuria. Microalbuminuria is a result of structural and functional transformational changes in the glomeruli.

Increased permeability is associated also with all other vessels in CVD. This means that the presence of microalbuminaria (and reduced eGFR) is predictive of CVD complications, as well as renal status. If renal insufficiency is diagnosed, tighter BP control is required to reduce further damage.

Evidence shows that the presence of microalbuminuria in people with established CVD, diabetes, or hypertension (even without diabetes) is associated with an increased relative risk of all-cause mortality, myocardial infarctions and stroke.

**Reference:**

> Chaudry S Chronic Kidney Disease (CKD) Lancet. 2012 Jan 14; 379 (9811):165-80.

## 19.4 Other Types of CVD

There are other, less common, types of CVD:

**Peripheral arterial disease** is strongly linked with coronary heartdisease, because they both undergo the same pathophysiological process, namely atherosclerosis. Thus they require the same assessments, preventative measures, and treatment modalities. Peripheral arterial disease occurs almost as frequently in women as it does in men, and smoking appears to be even more strongly linked in women with this condition, than with coronary heart disease.

**Aortic aneurysm and dissection** – an abnormal dilatation of the aorta indicating a weakness in the wall of the artery which can rupture (aneurysm), or a tear within the inner layers of the wall of the aorta resulting in leakage of blood between the layers forcing them apart (dissection). These both carry very poor prognoses, and share similar risk factors with other, more common, forms of CVD.

**Congenital heart disease** - malformations may occur because of genetic abnormalities or damaging exposure to drugs, alcohol or tobacco during gestation.

**Rheumatic Heart Disease** - caused by Streptococcal bacteria – is no longer so common anymore in westernised countries. It is more prevalent in Africa and Asia.

Other causes, such as **cardiac tumours**, **valvular disorders**, **cardiomyopathies** and **cardiac intimal disorders** can cause significant CVD, but are not as susceptible to risk factor modification, and so are not the focus for the preventative programme presented in this manual.

**Reference:**
  ➢ Types of cardiovascular disease - World Health Organisation
    www.who.int/cardiovascular_diseases/en/cvd_atlas_01_types

## In Summary
- We have described the pathophysiology of atheroma formation and hypertension.

- We have explained the concept of end-organ damage and how to understand which, and how, specific major organs are affected.

## Appendix D

## 20. World Bank Classification of Countries

As of 1 July 2015, low-income economies were defined as those with a gross national income (GNI) per capita, calculated using the *World Bank Atlas* method, of $1,045 or less in 2014; middle-income economies are those with a GNI per capita of more than $1,045 but less than $12,736; high-income economies are those with a GNI per capita of $12,736 or more. Lower-middle-income and upper-middle-income economies are separated at a GNI per capita of $4,125.

The UK is a high income country. Russia previously an upper middle income country was now redefined as a high-income economy.

**Reference:**

➤ http://data.worldbank.org/news/2015-country-classifications

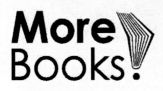

Printed by
**Schaltungsdienst Lange o.H.G., Berlin**